PELICAN BOOKS

THE EXPERIENCE OF CHILDBIRTH

Sheila Kitzinger was born in 1929 in Somerset. After obtaining her L.G.S.M. for teaching drama and voice production she studied social anthropology at Ruskin and St Hugh's College, Oxford, and did research and teaching at the University of Edinburgh.

Her B. Litt. thesis was on race relations in Britain, and her other studies have been of a group of English prostitutes and of the Rastafari sect in Jamaica. After nine months field research working in collaboration with the Medical Research Council at the University of the West Indies she is now writing a study of sex, pregnancy and childbirth amongst Jamaican women.

She has been preparing women for childbirth and developing her own Psychosexual Method since 1958, has been a leading member of the National Childbirth Trust since its foundation, lectured widely in North and South America, and has studied methods of childbirth education and the management of labour in various places as far afield as Mexico and East Germany. In 1971 she started to do research on the problems of West Indian women and their children in Britain, with an award from the Joost de Blank Research Fund.

She has been married to Uwe Kitzinger since 1952 and they live in Oxfordshire with their five daughters.

The photographs of the author in labour were taken by her husband.

The Experience of Childbirth

SHEILA KITZINGER

PENGUIN BOOKS

Penguin Books Ltd, Harmondsworth, Middlesex, England
Penguin Books Inc., 7110 Ambassador Road, Baltimore, Maryland 21207, U.S.A.
Penguin Books Australia Ltd, Ringwood, Victoria, Australia

—

First published in Great Britain by Victor Gollancz 1962
First published in the U.S.A. by Taplinger Publishing Co. Inc. 1972
Revised edition published in Pelican Books 1967
Reprinted with revisions 1970
Third edition 1972

—

Copyright © Sheila Kitzinger, 1962, 1967, 1972
Photographs copyright © Uwe Kitzinger, 1962

—

Made and printed in Great Britain
by C. Nicholls & Company Ltd
Set in Monotype Garamond

Contents

Acknowledgements

Above all I want to thank my husband for his constant encouragement and understanding, and for the way in which he has helped to make my own experience of childbirth among the happiest memories of our lives. It is to him that this book is dedicated.

My thanks also to *Medical World, New Society, The Spectator, The Nursing Mirror, The Teachers' Broadsheet* (National Childbirth Trust) and *Mother and Baby* for permission to absorb in the text articles of mine first published in their pages.

I am extremely grateful to Miss Chloe Fisher, S.R.N., S.C.M., M.T.D., a midwife of remarkable skill and sympathy, for working carefully through the first Pelican edition and making many helpful suggestions.

STANDLAKE MANOR
OXFORDSHIRE

Preface to the Pelican Edition

My two main lines of advance since the first edition was published have taken the form of a pincer movement; firstly to develop an entirely new approach to relaxation, using sensory memory, derived from Stanislavski acting techniques, including a new approach to awareness of the birth canal; and secondly to explore much further the psycho-sexual implications of pregnancy and birth in our society, and to integrate my relaxation techniques with the psycho-therapeutic potential of antenatal preparation, of which teachers have remained unaware for far too long. At the same time my teaching methods have developed a good deal; but doctors, midwives and others involved in the care of child-bearing women will find these discussed at length elsewhere.[1]

Here I have included many more detailed descriptions of the sensations of labour, written by women who have been my pupils and to whom I am deeply grateful for writing sometimes very lengthy and vivid accounts of their labours and of their feelings about the birth, the baby and the changed family. I think I have learned something from every single one of these hundreds who have given me their confidence.

It is sad that still so many women should embark upon childbirth in ignorance of their task in labour and with inadequate emotional preparation and support for the enormous physical and emotional changes involved. For far too many, pregnancy and birth is still something that happens *to* them rather than something they set out consciously and joyfully to do themselves.

Even attendance at 'relaxation' classes for expectant mothers does not necessarily mean that a woman is going to be given this sort of help. The quality of these classes varies throughout the country, and standards are only slowly being

1. Sheila Kitzinger, *An Approach to Antenatal Teaching*, National Childbirth Trust, London, 1967.

evolved and have no official recognition. Classes continue to be run in some hospitals by young and inexperienced physiotherapists who have never even seen a normal birth, let alone experienced any of the physical and emotional upheavals their pupils may be going through, and who have not had the additional training which the Obstetric Association of Chartered Physiotherapists claims is essential for antenatal work, or by midwives who sincerely believe that the best skills they can teach to mothers are the use of the gas-and-oxygen machine and plenty of 'mothercraft'.

But gradually things are changing. The Royal College of Midwives has publicly stressed the need for more antenatal education, and it only remains to be seen how this new educational skill of midwives is to be inculcated and developed and whether they are going to find time to take on the responsibilities involved.

The National Childbirth Trust of Great Britain is now creating a training scheme for antenatal teachers, which not only midwives and physiotherapists, but women who come from backgrounds other than these are also able to take.

It would be sheer waste not to use the skills which other trained women can bring to this kind of work; and the contribution of married women with children, who are, or were previous to marriage, teachers, sociologists, psychologists or nurses, for instance, and who can give up time for a course of study for a further professional qualification of this kind, can enrich and broaden this work.

More flexible methods of childbirth education are required, catering for example for the varying needs of different types of women, and taking into account not only the physiological functions of child-bearing, nor even only women's emotional states, but also the network of relationships and the particular culture within which they are caught up. We need not only a more psychologically oriented but also a sociologically oriented approach. The woman's expectations about birth, her role as a woman in any society, her early relationship with the baby, the effects of pregnancy and birth on the marriage and the wider family, the social environment within which a pregnant woman moves – all these are not simply matters of individual psychology but are essentially sociological phenomena. Even labour itself cannot really be exempted from sociological scrutiny.

For instance women even *feel* pain differently; and this is probably affected as much by social factors as by sheer physiology or by anything which might be uncovered by psychoanalytic techniques. Pain is always interpreted and placed within a predetermined scheme of things. In Jamaica I discovered that the West Indian peasant woman rarely feels discomfort on the perineum, or minds the pressure of the baby's head as it descends. But from case studies of English middle-class women it appears that many of them worry about dirtying the bed and are often shocked by sensations against the rectum and the vagina in labour – sensations which they may find excruciating. They feel distressed, in fact, at just those sensations which the peasant woman meets with equanimity. On the other hand the Jamaican peasant woman often anticipates and gets severe backache, a common enough experience all over the world. To her this pain is evidence of the back 'opening up' – which she believes it must do before the child can be born. So it looks as if cross-cultural and other sociological factors must be considered if we really want to understand what childbirth is all about.

Although you can show a woman how to have a baby just as she might learn how to make a soufflé, the whole thing may fall pretty flat at the last moment. Childbirth is not – and never has been – sheer obstetric dexterity and a hundred guineas to the magician who is doing it all for you. Nor is it an intellectual exercise for which you sit through a course soaking up academic information; after all, a great many women who don't know their pelvis from their perineum have borne their babies easily and with all the thrill of achievement. Nor is it an athletic performance for which one needs muscles like a boxer's biceps or an abdominal wall like the kitchen table. Nor simply a matter of squatting down amongst the leaves with the squirrels and little wild creatures and having it 'naturally'; today's obstetric skills are too precious for both the mother and the baby to forgo for that particular chimera of the imagination. Somewhere, somewhere along the line, it is a matter of the woman's expectations about labour, her relations with her body and her feelings about child-bearing, her deepest hopes and fears, her relationship with her husband and her parents, her acceptance of a new role, and the way in which she coordinates all these emotions and relationships. Then even physical difficulties can frequently be surmounted and fall into the background within the total picture of psychosomatic harmony.

Preface to the 1970 Edition

I HAVE brought the book entirely up to date, making alterations describing hospital procedures where these differ from those common in 1967.

The reader will still find a great deal about home confinements, however. I have included this material because I feel that, given careful selection of cases suitable for domiciliary delivery, and given good antenatal care, easy communication and positive co-operation between midwives, G.P.s and consultants, home is still the right place for many – probably most – women to have their babies. The midwife can provide the personal attention, detailed observation, and constant support during pregnancy and childbirth which takes place within the natural context of the family. Progress in obstetric care does not necessarily mean recourse to ever larger gleaming hospitals and the use of ever more complicated machines. It is important in our desire for progress that we do not ignore the need for personal caring – for developing skills in human relationships and deeper understanding. The task of modern medicine is not only to save lives, but to save our sanity.

Signs of the Times

FACED with the world problem of over-population, it looks as if a book about birth is irrelevant, and somehow runs counter to the trends of contemporary challenges. But if a woman is only going to have a few children, or one, how much more desirable it is that she makes a good job of it! She will not get an opportunity to enjoy later births, or to learn from earlier mistakes. Preparation for childbirth and planning *how* you hope to have your baby is the corollary to contraception and planning *when* you want to have the baby.

The emphasis upon motherhood, and preparation for just one role among the variety available to women today, may also seem to run counter to women's liberation and the movement to free women from the shackles of domesticity. But this is not the case: rather, the reverse. I should like to see women able to choose freely whether or not to use their fertility, to have control over their own bodies, and to decide how many children they wish to have, when and under what conditions; and, having decided, to enter on the process with understanding, free of the fears and ignorance of the past, and able to participate in and enjoy childbearing as much – even if in a different way – as they now feel they have the right to enjoy sex.

Bodies are for feeling with, and for actively living through and enjoying. When the healthy human body is engaged in a natural physiological process the individual normally feels pleasure and content: we enjoy eating and drinking and defecating, settling down to sleep and waking refreshed, walking and swimming, breathing the sea air and making love. In both repose and activity, in relaxation and effort, harmonious and co-ordinated physical functioning brings sensations of well-being. It used to be thought slightly vicious for women to feel anything very much in sexual intercourse except a gentle pleasure that they were loved and could please their husbands (or, at least, whatever the reality,

this was the sort of thing that found its way into print).
Women now expect to engage in sex actively, to have their
feelings studied by their partners, and to be made love to with
consideration and expertise so that they attain orgasm and
release. A whole crop of books and films, numerous appliances,
and pills and lotions have appeared on top of the counters
guaranteeing to bring success. It is all rather pathetic, as if
ecstasy could somehow be prescribed by using vaginal cream,
or by adopting the posture on page twenty-six instead of the
one on page thirty-two of the sex manual. It is almost as if
we are all trying to make up for lost time and to get in our
quota of sex and satisfaction before the curtains come down.

But sexuality is not simply a matter of coitus, or even of
what you do in bed. It certainly is not for a woman, and I
doubt whether it is for a man either. Currently accepted
definitions of sexuality are often crude and limited, and in
fact sexual skills need not be reduced to those culminating
in coitus. A woman's psychosexual life encompasses the
processes of childbearing, including pregnancy, birth,
commitment to the baby, feeding and touching it, the touching of bodies – all sorts of bodies, babies' and children's and
other people's – and the way she feels and thinks about her
body. The way a woman feels about her pregnancy and birth,
her whole manner of approaching it, and the way she behaves,
are part of her idea of herself as a woman and part of her
sexual nature.

Now women are looking at childbirth and wondering if
they have not been missing out on something. Maybe it is not
so much a curse laid upon Eve, a path of suffering to be trod
in order to have the joy of children, an occasion of shame
and humiliation and unmentionable practices down the lower
end of the body, as an exciting challenge, rewarding in itself,
and not simply as a means to an end.

I remember a scene in my grandmother's house when I was
a child. I must have been about seven. The aunts and grown-
up cousins were in the sitting room, and as I passed the seed
cake politely from one to the other I heard cousin Gladys
whisper to my mother that cousin Rose was expecting a baby.

The conspiracy of woman over the tea-cups and the hushed tones in which the information was conveyed told me that this was special and rather shocking news. Later on that day I shared my precious secret with another, younger, cousin. She was disbelieving – I cannot remember whether it was because Rose was not married, or whether she did not have a gooseberry bush, or the stork had not visited – but she asked, 'How can they *know*?', and I, having pored over my mother's midwifery books, unfortunately told her. I got into dreadful trouble about it and was obviously considered a contaminating influence. I felt unclean for a long time after. And I do not remember that carefully brought up little cousin ever being left alone with me again.

This was not in the Dark Ages (although it makes me feel part of history), but the casual way in which the story can be told now contrasts strongly with the crimson rush of shame I felt on being found out. I hope Rose enjoyed having her baby, though I doubt it. Anyway, she obviously stayed in the back of my mind, and the sense of childish outrage and injustice perhaps acted as a spur to doing something about women's ideas about childbirth, and towards creating the opportunity for women to give birth with awareness, understanding and delight.

I hope that the way many women look at childbirth now, the feelings of disgust, the fears and worries that they often have, even today, and the treatment often accepted as perfectly normal and to be expected in some antenatal clinics and hospitals, the all-too-real 'solitary confinements', the sceptical query 'Are you another of those relaxers? We don't believe in that here', and the women themselves who believe they are happier if they do not know 'too much', or who expect other people to get the baby born for them without any thought or preparation on their part – that in another thirty-five years all this will look equally out of date.

1971   S. K.

CHAPTER I

Childbirth With Joy

THE experience of bearing a child is central to a woman's life. Years after the baby has been born she remembers acutely the details of her labour and her feelings as the child was delivered. One can speak to any grandmother about birth and almost immediately she will begin to talk about her own labours. It is unlikely that any experience in a man's life is comparably vivid.

When women have suffered in childbirth – have felt humiliated and degraded by pain, through being the passive instruments of physical processes they could not understand – it is not only they who are affected. They carry with them through their lives the memory of this experience and by their attitude towards child-bearing affect other women and men – not only their own daughters and sons, but many others with whom they come into contact.

Pain in labour is real enough. We dare not underestimate the agony that some unprepared women endure in childbirth. It is not to be lightly glossed over by those more fortunate. Whether or not childbirth, as a natural function of the female body, 'should' be light and easy, it cannot be denied that for a great many women it is not. One woman described to me the intensely unpleasant sensations of delivery, and added that she had gritted her teeth so hard during the second stage that she had chipped off a front tooth. It can hardly be expected that a woman who goes through that sort of experience feels positively about child-bearing or can help a young pregnant woman to feel a joyful anticipation of the great adventure that confronts her.

But when a woman has her baby happily she spreads a different spirit – a mood of gladness rather than the dread and horror that is associated with most 'old wives' tales' and the gory accounts of labour which many women are able to produce for the benefit of expectant mothers.

It is this spirit of hope, this joy in birth as a fulfilment of a man and woman's love for each other, that should be the essence of childbirth – childbirth in which a woman finds delight in the rhythmic harmony of her body's functioning. Without this spirit perfect mechanical action in labour is not only made more difficult of attainment, but, even if achieved, is strangely unsatisfying.

Methods aiming at 'painless childbirth' deserve to be more widely understood. But the concern of this book, over and above that, is with a more positive experience. It is childbirth with joy.

THE PIONEERS

The history of the 'natural childbirth' movement has been one of unfortunate though perhaps inevitable conflict – not only between those who believed in its value and others who felt that it was all pointless, but between exponents of different theories. The philosophical bases upon which the different techniques are built are often incompatible, and in addition there is still a good deal of dispute as to the origins of the various endeavours to educate women for childbirth. It is probably a mistake to look for a single evolution of ideas and methods, and from the history of the movement it would appear that there has been spontaneous and independent development in different countries over the last twenty years.

Concern over the emotional adjustment of women in labour was first expressed by Grantly Dick-Read in the thirties.[1] His books, combined with the advances in obstetric physiotherapy stemming largely from the work of Helen Heardman, which in its turn owed a lot to that of Kathleen Vaughan and Minnie Randall, form the basis of most of the sorts of preparation for childbirth which many midwives and obstetricians in Britain

1. Grantly Dick-Read, *Introduction to Motherhood*, Heinemann, 1950; *Childbirth without Fear*, Heinemann, 1951; *Ante-natal Illustrated*, Heinemann, 1955.

today accept as smoothing the path of the woman in labour. Dick-Read's ideas and methods, however, have usually been very much diluted by the time they reach the pregnant woman visiting her antenatal clinic.

Methods used in Soviet hospitals[1] and based on Pavlovian techniques (those of the Pavlov who did the research on salivating dogs) are claimed as the chief inspiration of the French method called at first, unwisely, *accouchement sans douleur*, but now known – as in this country – as psychoprophylaxis. Though its French exponents had read their Dick-Read too, they claim that their approach is different in that it is based on building up a series of conditioned reflexes which in effect raise the pain threshold, so that sensations formerly interpreted by the brain as painful are accepted as painless. It was Fernand Lamaze, a French obstetrician working in a Communist trade union clinic in a grimy *quartier* of Paris, who on a visit to the Soviet Union was impressed by the calm in maternity wards practising these methods, brought them back with him to Western Europe, and invented new techniques – notably the 'panting like a dog' method of riding over contractions.[2] These methods which came largely from France and the U.S.S.R. have tended to emphasize the lack of painful sensations, but have, perhaps to the cost of some of those mothers who have adopted them, neglected that exhilaration which comes in a creative experience of completely harmonious psycho-physical functioning, where pain may or may not occur in the background – but if so, is willingly experienced as something that can be controlled, or else is brushed aside as being not nearly so important as the business of having a baby.

1. I. Velvovsky, K. Platonov, V. Ploticher and E. Shugom, *Painless Childbirth through Psychoprophylaxis,* Foreign Languages Publishing House, Moscow, 1960.

2. Fernand Lamaze, *Painless Childbirth,* Burke, 1958 (first published in French 1950). Pierre Vellay, *Childbirth without Pain,* Hutchinson, 1959. A somewhat different psychoprophylactic approach is described by S. Bazelaire and R. Hersilie in *Maternité,* La Table Ronde, 1963. The quarterly *Revue de médecine psychosomatique,* Librairie Maloine, regularly reports on more recent developments.

Mothers who have imagined that their labours would be completely painless have often suffered an unpleasant shock, and a woman not prepared for the powerful sensations and the astonishing force of uterine contractions may easily panic and be worse off than if she had had no instruction at all.

We have a very grave responsibility if a woman is trained for childbirth only to feel that she has failed at the first real pain. Most women must expect half an hour or so of pain or great discomfort at the end of the first stage.

THE ACTIVE ROLE OF THE MOTHER

If pain is great the mother can, of course, be anaesthetized, and pain-relieving drugs should always be available. There is nothing discreditable about accepting help as and when needed. Obstetricians may be reluctant to subject the child who is being born to large doses of drugs. Few mothers are able to look back upon their labours and say, as did Queen Elizabeth when she opened a new building of the Royal College of Obstetricians and Gynaecologists, 'You have given almost literal meaning to Wordsworth's assertion that "Our birth is but a sleep and a forgetting".'[1] Moreover, many women, far from welcoming the opportunity, do not like the idea of facing what are perhaps the most important moments of their lives completely unconscious. It is for this reason as much as because of the risks attendant upon the use of anaesthesia that Dr Guttmacher's account of modern childbirth as practised in the U.S.A. seems to me to make sad reading:

In favourable cases, under the influence of the drug triad, the patient falls into a deep quiet sleep between pains, but groans and moves about in a restless manner with each pain. The somnolent state continues into the second stage of labour and frequently for several hours after delivery. When the patient awakes, the obstetrician is rewarded by hearing her ask, 'Doctor, when am I going to have my baby?' The quickest way I know to prove that the child is already born is to have her feel her own abdomen. A newly restored waistline soon convinces even the most sceptical.[2]

1. As reported in The *Guardian*, 16 July 1960.
2. *Having a Baby,* Signet, U.S.A., 1950.

There are now available, of course, forms of regional anaesthesia – caudals, peridurals and epidurals involving spinal injections – which mean that the woman need neither have general anaesthesia and be 'out for the count', nor be so heavily doped that she is unable to concentrate on breathing and relaxing with contractions. The relatively new types of regional anaesthesia are sometimes spoken of as if they ought to be used for all women in childbirth, regardless of their inclinations, the amount of pain they are feeling, or what they have learned beforehand. Obstetricians often like them very much because the woman is perfectly controlled and rational, and is in no way overpowered by emotion or by the intensity of the labour experience. She often looks on like a more or less impartial observer of the scene, and he can get on with the task of delivering the baby. It is the sort of situation which fits in well with the routines of a busy hospital, and since the obstetrician almost invariably has to deliver with forceps or the vacuum-extractor, the delivery can be carefully timed and controlled, and be performed when he is on the spot and ready. Moreover if anything goes wrong with the uterine mechanism a synthetic hormone – syntocinon – can be used to initiate and control further contractions, without causing any discomfort to the mother. There have been cases of women reading a magazine while the obstetrician worked to deliver the baby down the other end! But in this very ease of manoeuvre lies a problem, or what some would see as a danger to the natural mechanisms. If the woman can feel nothing, or nothing painful, from the waist down, might it not be easier for all concerned if she received regional anaesthesia of this sort, however early on in labour, at the obstetrician's convenience, and then a syntocinon intravenous drip was inserted in her arm, and labour speeded up rapidly so that he could be available to deliver at a time suitable for him? This happens often in the U.S.A. and increasingly here. But however skilled at delivery the obstetrician is, and however well equipped the hospital with machines which record the baby's every heartbeat, with the instruments which can take a drop of blood from its scalp whilst still inside the uterus, and devices designed to make birth safer for the baby, patience still remains a virtue in midwifery, and nature is hurried overmuch at our peril. For this reason it is probably best to keep regional anaesthesia – which has obvious advantages when the woman is suffering pain – for cases for which it provides an evident solution to problems which cannot be met by the woman's own trained responses to uterine stimuli, or by emotional support and encouragement, which have an efficacy out of all proportion to their apparent significance.

Some women hope for regional anaesthesia – and this is especially so nowadays for epidurals – because in this way they feel they can co-operate with the birth process without having any discomfort. This is certainly true, but they may not realize that they may also be missing something – the intense and thrilling sensations of the descent of the baby's head, which can be not only painless, but enormously satisfying and enjoyable, even though at the same time it feels so extraordinary. Again and again I have heard women describe the keen sensuous pleasure they obviously experienced – and which often surprised them with its delight; it is not a question of just feeling the contractions and knowing when to push, but of the gradual opening up of the vagina like the uncurling petals of a rose. It may look as if it must be traumatic from the other end, and probably a good many of those attending in the delivery room are convinced that it must be painful for all women, and those who do not show it are simply the ones with better self-control; but this is not so. It can bring positive enjoyment, and precedes the sensations of delivery rather as intense sexual pleasure builds up to release in orgasm, and this – as tumultuously – even when it involves some pain.

It is not so much then the absence or deadening of pain which gives value to the method suggested in this book, but the addition of qualities which can make of childbirth a thrilling adventure, an achievement of the first order in which both husband and wife can share, and a revelation for both. I believe that in this sense childbirth should really be an experience through which we grow to greater spiritual and psychological fullness.

This involves the conscious participation of the woman. She is no longer a passive, suffering instrument. She no longer hands over her body to doctor and nurses to deal with as they think best. She retains the power of self-direction, of self-control, of choice, of voluntary decision and active cooperation with doctor and nurse. This involves a certain degree of intelligence[1] and knowledge of the processes of pregnancy and labour. She must also have a mind which is not only relatively free of fear but filled with pleasurable anticipation of labour. To achieve the rhythmic coordination and harmony which is the essence of a beautifully controlled labour she must above all, *have learned to trust her body and her instincts*. We are seeking to achieve a functional harmony of the woman's body which to a few civilized women comes naturally, but which most of us have to learn painstakingly through the months of pregnancy.

Some people think that 'natural childbirth' implies a sort of hypnotic relation between the doctor and patient and that unless a patient is unusually suggestible this method will fail for her. Nothing could be farther from the truth. A woman who is adequately prepared can find this method works well even if the obstetrician or midwife knows nothing about it at all; all she requires is that they shall be permissive, and, ideally, that her husband shall be present and willing and able to take responsibility and to cooperate with the other members of the labour team, since she should not get involved in explanation at this time.

All this necessitates a definite commitment at some stage during the first half of pregnancy, a positive decision to undertake preparation for labour and a willingness to learn. Often a woman has to seek far before she can find the sort of instruction she requires, since it is not given in every hospital and

1. It has been reported from France that 'intellectual women do better in labour than those who are factory workers, domestic servants, etc.' See Claude Revault-d'Allonnes, 'Une enquête préliminaire sur l'accouchement sans douleur', *Revue française de sociologie*, I, No. 2, 1960.

clinic. A woman cannot stumble into this sort of childbirth without preparation. Quite often women have quick or easy labours without any previous instruction, as every midwife and obstetrician knows, but even quick and easy labours do not bring the fullness of joy which comes from a labour in which a woman has been, despite possible pain, co-operating with understanding.

The end result of this preparation during pregnancy is not athletic skill, super-elastic muscles or the ability to breathe like a Yogi and relax until one is in a hypnotic stupor, but a mental state, an emotional preparedness without which no amount of physical exercise can effect adequate preparation for the experience of labour.

This was the basis of Grantly Dick-Read's emphasis upon fearlessness and the clearing away of psychological obstructions so that a woman could have her baby as nature intended. However much we have extended and elaborated our skills in training for childbirth, we cannot afford to lose the spirit that shone through Dick-Read's courageous work in the early days when the whole subject seemed suspect to many of the established leaders of the medical profession.

I am aware that some people find all mystical notions about childbirth particularly unacceptable, and certain of Dick-Read's most sincerely felt statements of a metaphysical kind brought him into disrepute with some who prided themselves on their practical natures. I would not suggest that one should approach childbirth borne on the wings of a pseudo-mysticism which might collapse at the crucial moment; nevertheless, to anyone who thinks about it long enough, birth cannot simply be a matter of techniques for getting a baby out of one's body. It involves one's relationship to life as a whole, the part one plays in the order of things; and as the baby develops and can be felt moving inside, to some women annunciation, incarnation, seem to become facts of their own existence.

DIFFERENT METHODS OF RELAXATION

Physical preparation is, however, important, and relaxation forms its basis, the prerequisite without which a happy labour is unlikely. And yet there is a good deal of misunderstanding as to what this relaxation really means. One should in fact carefully distinguish three types of relaxation, any one or a combination of which may be encountered in antenatal classes today.

Firstly, in many hospitals and clinics relaxation is still taught as a kind of 'flopping' and women are urged to let their thoughts wander and to day-dream and think about beautiful things, not focusing their minds upon anything, while the midwives go off to make everyone a cup of tea. This sort of relaxation, useful as it may be in everyday life – and even then we cannot always have the seclusion and the time in which to practise it – presents its own perils for the woman in labour. The auto-suggestion that she is required to use to get into this state is so far removed from the reality of the situation – the great muscle of the uterus grinding away like a tremendous dynamo, the stretching of other muscles, the movements of the baby as he sinks lower, the never-ceasing activity going on within her and usually also around her – that, unless she manages to withdraw from her labour entirely and enter into a state of amnesia, labour is going to be a cruel shock. Even if she succeeds in becoming so amnesic that she does not register pain, she cannot be a fully responsive and cooperative patient, and she runs the risk of an uncontrolled delivery. But in fact many mothers who try to drift away from the sensations of labour, and who have never been made aware of the intensity of the feelings they will experience, are unable to escape and are threatened by severe pain once the contractions get really powerful. It is only too easy once this has happened to lose one's confidence, to be submerged under waves of contractions, and to try to turn and run from one's ordeal or simply to give in and suffer.

Secondly, Dick-Read taught relaxation based on the Jacobson method of progressive relaxation;[1] Jacobson's method

1. Jacobson, *Progressive Relaxation,* University of Chicago Press, 1939.

involves a careful analysis of the nature of contractions in different muscle groups – muscles which normally act in unison with each other when one turns one's head to one side, for instance – so that the person doing it understands exactly which ones are doing the work, and learns to alternately contract and release them completely. Psychoprophylaxis took this same method but emphasized Jacobson's differential relaxation and invented exercises for the limbs which they called 'disassociation'. An exercise of this kind involves, for instance, contracting all the muscles of the right arm, while the rest of the body remains relaxed, or contracting muscles of the right arm and leg, or left arm and leg, while other muscles are 'decontracted'. A woman able to do these exercises well is doubtless very efficient at controlling tension in her body under the conditions imposed by the exercise sessions; it does not mean, however, that she can relax in situations of stress, and, anyway, she is not required to perform drills of this kind in labour. So such exercises can become something in the nature of conjuring tricks – great fun to do perhaps, but not very useful. In situations of stress we tend to spontaneously contract muscle groups which act together, which do not correspond to 'all down the left side' or 'both arms' or 'one arm and the leg on the other side', as in these exercises, and working with muscles in groups which quite naturally act in sympathy with each other – as Jacobson suggested – is probably more relevant to the labour situation. But both these methods are a great advance over the 'dream you're floating on a cloud' type of approach.

The method described in Chapter 4 of this book, though also partly indebted to Jacobson, differs from all these, and owes a great deal to the 'Method' school of acting and also to experiments in touch and massage, which I first began to develop three or four years ago when working with husbands and wives together, some of whom were going through particularly difficult phases in their marriage, and which were given added impetus by my visit to the U.S.A. in 1970. During a lecture tour I also met people who had been working at Esalen, and we discovered that in some respects we were working along similar lines. Since then I have been using my method of 'Touch Relaxation' with older women facing problems of tension, too, and with couples encountering psychosexual problems.

THE EMOTIONS OF CHILDBIRTH

'Natural childbirth' has meant many different things and has covered every degree of training from the most intensive to the most rudimentary and fragmentary of morale-boosting (with a definite tendency towards the latter). In fact it is only confusing to label all these different types of preparation with the single term of 'natural childbirth'. When I first began teaching such techniques I was more interested in easily identifiable and measurable results which could be observed in a labour and recorded on a case sheet. To me, then, a tear or a prolonged labour meant that I had failed with that case, and whilst I was pleased to hear women speak happily about their labours I was more concerned to analyse the accounts with which they presented me in order to arrive at the selected criteria which obstetric medicine has tacitly accepted as relevant to the evaluation of the success or failure of methods used in childbirth.

These criteria are concerned, however, solely with the physical machine involved in parturition. They can, indeed, give us some idea of what labour was like for the women having the babies, but sometimes – much more often than we take for granted – they are very far off the mark in giving any indication of the emotional experience which the women had. Particularly is this true regarding the total length of labour and length of the first and second stages; long labours can be pleasant and brief labours can sometimes be unpleasant.

Physiological criteria are not the only factors which should be considered in evaluating a woman's labour. The really important thing about a labour – apart from the one which we are in no danger of underestimating, of having a live mother and a live baby – is how the woman copes with it, and how she emerges from the experience – the effect it has on her mind.

This is as much a matter for serious scientific inquiry as are all the physiological criteria which are usually applied; a woman's feelings about her labour – whether or not they appear to correspond to reality – are just as relevant, even if they must be analysed by rather different techniques. We are dealing here with two orders of reality – the physical facts and the psychological facts. In any labour they are intertwined with and act and react upon each other.

A leading obstetrician once remarked to me on the extent to which many women misrepresented their labours. One woman in his hospital was talking about her two previous frightful labours, and was elaborating accounts of the complicated manoeuvres to which the obstetrician had recourse 'to get it away'. From interest he looked up her records, and discovered, he said, that she had had two spontaneous births. He felt that this shows how untruthful women were liable to be. I was more interested in the state of mind of a woman who wanted to believe that she had had difficult births. Is it not likely that, however easy these births were from the doctor's point of view, for her they were difficult? Denied the justification of her emotional upheaval by reference to accompanying physical difficulties, perhaps she was forced to invent these physical complications. Only then was her emotional distress justifiable.

On the other hand, a woman having an apparently bad labour who seems physically near the end of her tether can yet say, in the middle of that labour, 'It's wonderful'. This is something which we do not yet fully understand. It has been suggested that it is a form of 'sub-hypnosis'; but since to the layman this immediately suggests that the woman is in a state of semi-trance, and that she is subject to the influence of another person, the removal of whose presence would result in the obliteration of the state of euphoria by pain and distress, the term is misleading. For this is, in fact, not the case.

With whatever a woman's contentment and true peace in labour is associated, and whatever name we give it, this is something that cannot be left out of the reckoning. It would be a strange materialism which evaluates the birth according to purely physical standards unrelated to the state of mind of the woman who is bearing the child. A woman is not just a machine through which a baby is brought to birth by the doctor or midwife, a convenient receptacle for the developing foetus in pregnancy, a receptacle which at the time of labour offers more or less resistance to the child's entry into the world, and which is judged fit or wanting according to the efficient functioning of its parts. This efficiency is important, of course, but the body is part of a *person* for whom the birth of the baby is of major emotional significance. It is the aim of this book to help parents make childbirth an experience faced with serenity and joy and to gain from it a sense of achievement and a deep, shared happiness.

CHAPTER 2

Pregnancy

FERTILIZATION

FERTILIZATION occurs when the male sperm buries itself inside the wall of one of the female *ova*, or eggs, which grow in pockets inside the ovaries. The ova are the largest cells in the human body, but even so they are only 0·2 millimetres in diameter. Each month a ripe ovum is freed from the ovary and starts a journey along the uterine tube towards the uterus. Unless it meets a sperm, it is expelled still unfertilized, but if it becomes fertilized it stays in the uterus and grows into a baby.

The male sperms grow inside the testicles and are ejaculated into the woman's vagina in the semen. Each sperm has a flattened oval head and a long lashing tail, rather like a miniature tadpole, and is between 52 and 62 thousandths of a millimetre long.

Once the ovum is fertilized it starts to segment until it is a mass of tightly packed cells called the *morula*, like a blackberry. The outer ones are called the *trophoblast* and form a container for the inner ones which create the embryo.

Liquid is formed between these two sorts of cells. The inside section of the inner cells (the *endoderm*) now turns into a yolk-sac, and then this endoderm separates from the outer layer (*ectoderm*), each drawing aside from the other, and a third layer of germ cells (the *mesoderm*) is formed between them. The outside layer forms the baby's nervous system, the outer layer of the skin, the sweat glands, oil glands and mammary glands, the hair, nails, nose, mouth, eyes, and some other organs. The inside layer forms the digestive tract and glands, the auditory tubes, lungs, bladder and parts of the thyroid and thymus glands. The middle layer forms the skeleton, muscles, circulatory system and some other parts of the body.

By the end of the third week after fertilization, two

longitudinal folds have formed in the outside layer, called the neural folds, with the dip between them called the neural groove. The groove gets progressively deeper and the folds close over it to make a tube, the neural tube, and where the baby's brain will be there appear three bumps, the sites of the forebrain, midbrain and hindbrain. The long part of the tube forms the spinal cord.

Along the front of the neural tube a thick ridge grows (the *notochord*), from the future midbrain right down to where the vertebral column will later grow.

Toward the end of the second week after fertilization the middle layer of cells begins to divide to form later the skeleton of the trunk.

A part of the yolk-sac is embedded in the embryo at the umbilicus. The embryo is enclosed within a sac of membranes and floats in *amniotic fluid* – clear, colourless and sterile water – which at the same time protects it and allows it to move.

After about a week in the uterine tube the fertilized ovum reaches the uterus and buries itself in the lining. (It is this lining which was released every month in the menstrual period.) The outside layer of cells of the embryo throws out tentacles known as *villi* which dig into the walls of the uterus and get nutrition for the developing embryo from them. At first these *villi* cover the whole outer layer of cells, but after the end of the second month they atrophy, except at the site of the placenta.

THE FUNCTION OF THE PLACENTA

It is through the placenta that the foetus is nourished, is oxygenated and can excrete its waste after the first two months of pregnancy. The thin walls of the *villi* separate the foetal bloodstream from the mother's blood, but the foetus absorbs oxygen and nutrition through them and can excrete its waste material through their delicate walls. Although the baby gets its oxygen and is fed through the mother's bloodstream, there is no direct passage of blood between the mother and the baby or the baby and the mother. The baby is nourished by her through a process of *osmosis* – that is, certain constituents of the mother's blood percolate through to the baby. Many substances which would be harmful to the baby are sieved off in this way so that they never reach him. The placenta usually lies at the top of the uterus. The umbilical cord connects the foetus to the placenta, and is attached somewhere near the middle. Because the cord is made of slippery jelly, and the baby is floating in liquid, true knots in the cord are extremely rare, and it is frequently twisted around the child's neck without doing any harm. Neither the baby nor the mother can feel anything in this cord, since no nerve supply runs through it. After the birth of the baby the placenta is expelled and the openings of the torn uterine vessels are shut by contraction of the muscle fibres of the uterine walls. By this time the placenta is a disc-shaped mass with a diameter of from 7 to 8 inches, a thickness at the middle of about $1\frac{1}{4}$ inches, and weighs about 1 lb. It looks like a large piece of raw liver.

THE PELVIS

The pelvic girdle is formed by the hip-bones, which create a shape something like a lobster-pot sloping downwards and forwards, through which the baby passes when he is being born. The pelvic outlet is limited by the *sub-pubic arch* in front, the *ischial tuberosities* at the sides and the *sacrum* behind. The *coccyx*, the little bone at the bottom of the spine, although curved forward, is attached to the sacrum by a joint which moves back when the baby is being born, so that it does not get in the way.

Most pelves present no difficulties in childbirth and provide ample room for the baby. Prenatal examinations can indicate whether there is likely to be any problem with a malformed pelvis and a large baby. But usually the shape of the pelvis allows a straightforward labour.

THE UTERUS

The internal reproductive organs of a woman are composed of a hollow, thick-walled, muscular *uterus* or womb, shaped like a pear with the stalk end pointing downwards and usually slightly backwards. It is about 3 inches long. In front and behind are the bladder and the rectum, and the mouth of the uterus, or *cervix*, connects up with the vagina below. From the upper part of the uterus two tubes or *oviducts* run towards the small almond-shaped *ovaries* which lie on either side.

By the end of pregnancy the uterus has moved up out of the pelvis into the abdomen, and is marrow-shaped and about 12 inches long. Its *fundus* (the top) is nearly as high as the *diaphragm*, which is the sheet of muscle which separates the abdomen from the *thorax* (chest). The baby is protected within the walls of the uterus, which are about half an inch thick, and is also inside a bag of membranes, where he floats in a sea of *liquor*[1] *amnii* (the 'waters'), attached by the umbilical cord to his placenta, through which he is nourished.

THE DEVELOPMENT OF THE FOETUS

The dating of pregnancy is usually reckoned in relation to the first day of the last menstrual period – when the baby was still not conceived!

Three weeks: The ovum is the size of a small grape. No human characteristics can be recognized.

Four weeks: The sac is 1″ long, about the size of a pigeon's egg. The embryo measures about ⅜″. It is curved like a broad bean so that head and tail almost meet. The rudimentary eyes are visible and small buds indicate where limbs will develop.

Eight weeks: The sac is the size of a hen's egg. The placenta begins to grow. The embryo is slightly over 1″ long. Hands and feet are recognizable. The head is large in proportion to the body. The heart, which will work for a life-time, has begun to beat.

1. The first syllable rhymes with 'hike'.

Twelve weeks: The sac is the size of a goose's egg and the placenta, which is now well formed, weighs more than the foetus. The length of the foetus is $3\frac{1}{2}''$ and it weighs just under 2 oz. Fingers and toes are evident.

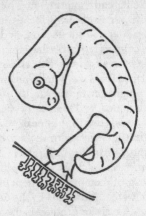

Sketch of the embryo at about a month old. At this stage the developing embryo still looks much like a baby seahorse. It is about 10 mm. long. Notice the eye, the rudimentary limbs, nose and mouth.

Sixteen weeks: The foetus measures 6″ and weighs approximately 6 oz. Foetal movements are present; sex can be distinguished. *Meconium* is present in the intestine. This is the baby's first stool. It is very dark green and is expelled from the bowel during the first few days after birth.

Twenty weeks: The foetus is 8″ long and weighs 10 oz. *Vernix caseosa* – a substance very much like cold cream or cottage cheese – is present on the skin and helps to protect it. It may or may not be present at birth. There are fine downy hairs on the head, and eyebrows. Finger-nails can be distinguished. Foetal movement is felt by the mother (quickening) and the foetal heart can be heard.

Twenty-four weeks: The foetus measures 12″ and weighs about $1\frac{1}{2}$ lb.

Twenty-eight weeks: The foetus measures 14″ and weighs 2½ lb. Legally, the foetus is viable but only 2 to 4 per cent of these very immature babies live.

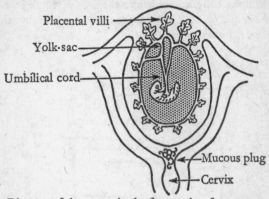

Placental villi

Yolk·sac

Umbilical cord

Mucous plug

Cervix

Diagram of the uterus in the first weeks of pregnancy.

Thirty-two weeks: The foetus measures 16″ and weighs 3½ lb. The skin is red and wrinkled. Fine downy hairs – which are called *lanugo* – are on the baby's body. About 40 to 50 per cent of babies born at this stage survive.

Thirty-six weeks: The foetus is 18″ long and weighs 5½ lb. There is a little subcutaneous fat. The nails reach the finger tips and the cartilage of the ears is soft. The survival rate is good. About 94 per cent can be reared if suitable care is given.

Forty weeks: The foetus measures 20″ and weighs 7 lb. The baby is well covered with subcutaneous fat and the skin is red but not wrinkled.

The woman begins to feel her baby moving at any time between sixteen and twenty weeks, usually early with second and subsequent babies, as she already knows what it feels like. Some women say it feels like butterflies; some think it is more like goldfish swimming round; others feel a soft thudding or something akin to a slight electric shock. It is more noticeable when the mother relaxes, and especially when she lies down at night and is about to go to sleep.

During pregnancy the uterus rises out of the pelvis into the abdomen, and by about 34 or 36 weeks is right up under the mother's ribs. The fuller the uterus, the higher it is likely to rise, until the baby descends into the pelvis. Hence in a twin pregnancy the *fundus* – or top of the uterus – is higher than it would be expected to be.

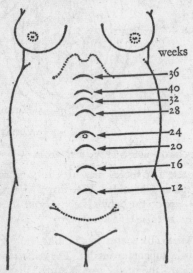

Diagram showing the approximate height of the fundus at various stages in pregnancy. Notice the descent after the baby has engaged.

Variation in birth weight is considerable and anything between 6 and 10 lb. is normal. To be on the safe side in most hospitals babies under 5 or 5½ lb. are treated as premature, whether or not born at term. But a baby's maturity – that is, whether or not it is born at full term – can be more important than its weight.

THE PHYSIOLOGY OF LABOUR

When labour starts, rhythmically recurring contractions of the uterus gradually thin out or 'efface' and then dilate the cervix, which is already soft as a result of hormone activity. These

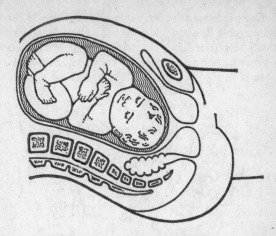

THE BABY BEFORE LABOUR BEGINS

The baby will probably turn slightly towards the mother's back in order to enter the brim of the pelvis.

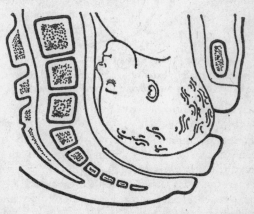

THE DELIVERY OF THE BABY: I

In the second stage the baby's head is flexed forward on his chest as he descends the birth canal, the shape of which causes the head to rotate, and the occiput (the crown of the head) is in an anterior position so that the baby is facing the mother's back. As the head reaches the pelvic floor the perineum starts to bulge forward.

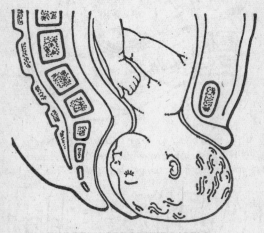

THE DELIVERY OF THE BABY: 2

The birth of the head by extension. The baby's head crowns. Notice that the baby's chin is now lifted well up off his chest.

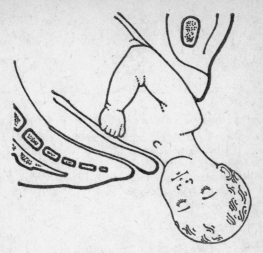

THE DELIVERY OF THE BABY: 3

The baby's head slips out and then it starts to turn to come into line with the shoulders which are still inside. It passes through approximately a right-angle. This is called 'external rotation' and 'restitution'. It all happens quite naturally without assistance. The baby's skin is of a purplish-blue colour.

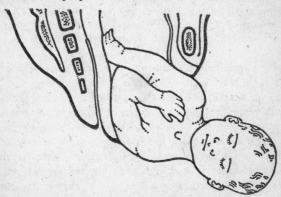

THE DELIVERY OF THE BABY: 4

The anterior shoulder (i.e. the one nearest the mother's abdomen) is usually delivered first. Then the rest of the baby's body slides out.

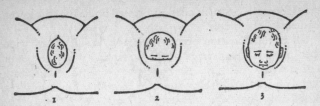

THE BIRTH OF THE BABY'S HEAD IN MORE DETAIL

1) The assistants and the father can see the baby's head at each contraction, but it disappears again between contractions. The perineum is being slowly and gently dilated.

2) The head crowns, and the mother may be able to look down and see it if she is in a suitable position.

3) The head oozes out.

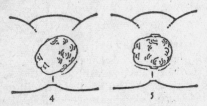

4) The head begins to rotate externally in order to come into line with the shoulders which are not yet born. This happens between contractions or at the start of the next contraction.

5) At this point the mother can see her baby's face for the first time.

contractions have been estimated to exert a pressure of about 30 lb. per square inch. The cervix is first drawn up and later pulled open and the lower segment stretched until the completion of the first stage of labour, by which time it has been completely dilated. This is by far the longest stage of labour and, with a woman having her first baby, usually takes between about six and thirteen hours, although some women are much quicker and some much slower, and some are not aware of the beginnings of dilatation. In the case of a heavy baby, labour may be a little longer. With subsequent babies labour is usually more rapid. The first stage may last from about four to about eight hours, but there is great variation. The baby's head,

flexed forwards on to his chest, is pressed down into the lower
segment of the uterus.

When full dilatation occurs the cervix is sufficiently wide
open to allow the passage of the presenting part (the head).
The cervix is the size of the palm of a man's hand including
the thumb joint – approximately 10 cm. or 5 inches. At
this point expulsive contractions, with or without the
voluntary help of the mother, have the effect of forcing the
baby down the birth canal. First the baby's head is pressed
down towards the mother's back in order to get through the
pelvic cavity. It is flexed even more and rotates at approximately a right angle. As the head reaches the pelvic floor muscles the perineum (the tissues around and between the anus and
the vagina) starts to bulge out, and internal rotation is complete. The head then passes beneath the pubic arch (*pubis
symphysis*). Then the perineum slips back over the face and
under the chin and the baby's head turns to come in line with
the shoulders which are still inside, rotating again through an
approximate right angle. The shoulder nearest the mother's
abdomen is usually born first, and then the other shoulder.
After this the baby's body slips out. The second stage usually
lasts from about a few minutes to about an hour – or occasionally two hours – and does not often last longer than about half
an hour with a woman having her second baby.

THE PELVIC FLOOR

The sheet of muscles across the floor of the pelvic cavity is
called the pelvic floor. These muscles are often used only unconsciously or involuntarily, in defecation and micturition
(passing water), and in sexual intercourse when a woman is
mounting to orgasm. Many women are not aware that they
possess them. It has been said that 'the term "floor" is not a
good one, since it leads one to think of the floor of a house,
e.g. a rigid partition running transversely between walls.
Consequently in looking for a floor in the pelvis we are apt
to seek for something which has the character of a house
floor. The pelvic floor has no such structure. It is not a rigid

partition, nor does it run transversely. It is elastic and mov-
able, varying in its thickness, its nature, and its slope at various
parts, while it runs across a very irregularly shaped space –
the outlet of the bony pelvis. It is composed of a variety of
tissues differing in their consistence, their strength, and the
firmness of their attachment to the bony wall.'[1]

These muscles forming the floor of the pelvis are even more
important than the muscles which form the wall of the abdomen. During early pregnancy and later, after the baby is born,
when a woman wants to get her figure back, she is very conscious of the abdominal wall and reminds herself to hold it in
and so strengthen the muscles which form a natural corset
around the abdomen. In my experience, with women who
prepare themselves for childbirth this usually comes quite
spontaneously. But there is far less awareness of the importance
of the muscles of the pelvic floor. Simply because they are not
seen they can very easily be forgotten. They are important
because they form a base to all the abdominal and pelvic vis-
cera and support the kicking, squirming baby *in utero* rather
like a trampoline. If they are allowed to get very lax and
strained the uterus can slip down out of place, often giving
a woman bad backache and making her tired and irritable in
the process, and can drop so low that it even protrudes into
the vagina. This is the prolapse of middle age, from which
younger women can also suffer. It occurs commonly after
any excessive straining, either with inefficient bearing-down
during labour, as a result of constant lifting of heavy objects without correct muscle-coordination, or as a result of
chronic constipation. In the past it was considered the almost
inevitable consequence of repeated child-bearing. This can be
remedied by exercise of the voluntary muscles in mild cases,
but if it is permitted to get very bad the only sure remedy is
surgery.

Helen Heardman[2] has likened muscle to elastic which, in-

1. Clarence Webster, *Researches in Female Pelvic Anatomy*, Young J.
Pentland, 1892.

2. *Relaxation and Exercise for Natural Childbirth*, Livingstone, 1956. *A
Way to Natural Childbirth*, Livingstone, 1948.

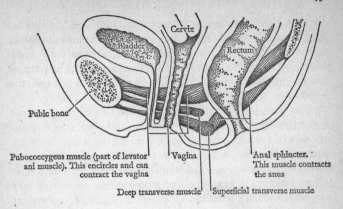

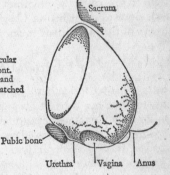

Pubic bone

Pubococcygeus muscle (part of levator ani muscle). This encircles and can contract the vagina

Vagina

Anal sphincter. This muscle contracts the anus

Deep transverse muscle

Superficial transverse muscle

A stylised view

Here the pelvic floor is seen as a muscular basin with an opening below at the front. The muscular tissues are supported by and enclosed in the pelvic bones shown hatched

PELVIC FLOOR[1]

Diagram to illustrate the position of muscles of the pelvic floor over which voluntary control can be obtained.

stead of losing its power to stretch and recoil by continued use, gains in tone as a result of constant exercise. The more muscles are used, the more able they are to retain the sort of tension which is necessary to support the internal organs, and the more complete the rehabilitation of the body after childbirth. On the other hand the 'muscle-bound' woman tends to suffer laceration during delivery and it is also important that

1. Slightly adapted from *Obstetrics Illustrated,* Gorrey, Govan, Hodge and Callander, Livingstone, 1969.

we should teach these particular muscles how to 'give'. They form the gateway through which a baby is born into the world, and open up as the head is descending; as the baby slides through the pelvic floor these structures are pulled apart as one might stretch the neck-band of a turtle-neck sweater into which one was wriggling. They do so more readily if the woman does not offer resistance to the baby's birth, and if she is sufficiently aware of their positions and their functions to know when she is contracting and releasing them. They are already in a more elastic and softer condition, as are many other tissues of the body, as a result of the action of hormones during pregnancy. Indeed, in some women they are so soft that they involuntarily pass water when they cough, sneeze or laugh. In this case it is important to practise exercises for the pelvic floor as described in Chapter 6 and to pull in all the muscles of the pelvic floor as one is about to cough.

HOME OR HOSPITAL?

A woman has to decide fairly early in pregnancy whether she wants to have her baby in hospital or at home. One would wish for both the safety of hospital and the comfort of home, but to some extent it is nowadays a choice between these alternatives. Having a baby is not like a surgical operation, and the woman's attitude of mind is all-important in the ease and spontaneity with which she can perform her function of giving birth. Unless there are reasons why it is best for the baby to be born in hospital (either medical or 'social' reasons, which include not having sufficient room), home is therefore often the best place to have the baby, but, of course, in those cases where difficulties are likely to crop up hospital is by far the safest place to be. Some women are unusually fearful of possible complications and of suffering unnecessary pain at home. Such psychological reasons for preferring hospital confinement must also be taken into account. It may be that as the expectant mother learns more about childbirth during her pregnancy she will come to feel more confident. She should book a hospital bed within the first three months, however, as it may be difficult to get one if she leaves it till mid-pregnancy.

It is worth remembering that in Britain a maternity grant of £22 is available and this helps with expenses. Having a baby at home need not be costly. The main expense involved in a home confinement is secondary to the birth itself and is connected with getting adequate domestic help for the period which used to be called 'lying in', and which nowadays means that period of time during which the mother is concentrating exclusively on herself and the baby and does not bother herself with housework or unnecessary cooking. A home help should be obtainable through one's Local Authority. It is quite possible to have a baby at home even without living-in domestic help if the husband can take a week off and is prepared to do some domestic chores, but even then one must reckon with additional expenses, including more expensive food, and laundry charges, since few husbands have the same ideas of domestic economy as their wives. If the couple plan to spend that time together in a leisurely holiday atmosphere, eating simply prepared food and not trying to follow a clock-work routine, they can thoroughly enjoy each other with their new baby.

SOME OF THE ADVANTAGES OF HAVING A BABY AT HOME

Perhaps one of the most important reasons for having a home confinement is that the mother is in the security of an environment with which she is familiar and which she likes. The whole process seems more natural than it can do in hospital and she is far less likely to be frightened. Labour appears to be shorter, since she does not commit herself to it so early, but carries on with her normal activities. She has privacy – something which many women value highly and which, unless she is in a private room, she cannot have in hospital. As a result it may be easier to adopt the method described in this book at home rather than in hospital (although there exist some progressive units which are shining exceptions), where one has the concentrated individual care of a midwife whom one already knows. The husband – if he is wise – will also have met the midwife, and they can work together as a team. An additional, and to many women not inconsiderable, advantage with home confinement is that the woman is not left alone during her labour. Someone, either the midwife or the husband, is always with her. There are no difficulties about the husband being present to help his wife at home, whereas there are in many hospitals, and the future parents should always inquire about hospital protocol in this matter, since in some hospitals it is still never permitted.

Contrary to general opinion, I think that as compared with hospital the mother at home probably has more peace and quiet. She is not troubled by the events and distress of any other woman's labour, as she may be in hospital. She usually gets more opportunity to sleep and to relax after the birth, since there is no hospital schedule to be rigidly followed (some sort of routine is necessary in every institution). She is treated as an individual and is not expected to conform to a pattern for the ease of running of a large and often ill-planned and under-staffed ward. She can have her baby with her, can cuddle him when she likes and feed him whenever he wants, and can get to understand him; she can see that he is not given sugared water – which may satisfy his thirst without stimulating the supply of breast milk by his repeated sucking, and which encourages a lazy feeder to be even sleepier when offered the breast. He is not left to cry, and, since his needs are immediately satisfied, tends to be more peaceful than the hospital baby. The dangers of cross-infection are also avoided. These are very real in many maternity units.[1] The mother can move about when

1. R. Illingworth, *The Normal Child*, p. 132, Churchill, 1959: 'In a British hospital known to me 158 babies under 1 year of age were admitted to medical wards for treatment in the first 6 months of 1947. Of these 44 (27.8 per cent) acquired infections in hospital, and 8 died as a result of those infections. More than 5 per cent of the babies, therefore, who were admitted for treatment died of infections acquired in the hospital. . . . It is very difficult to compare accurately the incidence of infections in different maternity units, because the standard of accuracy in recording them varies so greatly. It seems clear however, from published work, annual reports and other sources that it is common for 10–20 per cent of all new-born babies to acquire infections – *most of them admittedly very trivial ones* – while in hospital.' [My italics.]

she feels like it and is not propped up in a sitting position in bed. (This immobility is a contributory factor in thrombosis.)

The father, too, has a much bigger share in the first days of the baby's life than if his wife were in hospital. He does not have to view his child through plate-glass, which remains the custom in some hospitals. He knows that he is necessary to his wife and child and is not treated as a germ-ridden intruder. The mother can see her friends and relatives when she likes instead of at set visiting times, and this, for some, is an additional, though less important, advantage.

But maybe the confusion of a home confinement is not really worth it? Some people think that the whole house needs to be reorganized in order to have a baby at home – but this is far from the truth, and district midwives do as little as possible to disrupt the normal running of the home. Forty years ago things were rather different, and those who considered they were taking adequate precautions against infection used to strip the room where the confinement was to take place of all hangings, curtains and carpets, remove all pictures, ornaments and books, and turn it into a sort of operating-theatre. Sometimes a sulphur candle would be burned in the room in order to sterilize it, and all the doors and windows were sealed to keep out germs and dust. When the woman was in labour the seals were broken and she lay on a high bed in the middle of the room with a board placed under the mattress to make it firm, and a roller towel strung round the bed-posts for her to pull and strain on.[1] After the baby was born she had to go on sleeping in her single bed and her husband was not allowed to sleep beside her. Often she had to lie flat for a number of hours or even days after the confinement, and was not allowed to get out of bed for a fortnight. For six weeks after she was still something of an invalid. She was tightly bound up in a binder or large towel wound round her abdomen because it was thought that this would help to get her figure back, but

1. This is bad because, besides exhausting the woman, it tends to make her concentrate on pulling with her arms rather than on pressing the baby out.

she was not permitted to do any exercises with this end in view.[1]

In an effort to breast-feed the baby she was urged to consume vast quantities of liquid and bottle after bottle of stout,[2] and often was allowed neither fruit nor vegetables, and certainly not salads as they were thought to give the baby wind. With lack of any form of muscular exercise and a poor diet she must very often have suffered from constipation, and, indeed, this was and still is by some people considered a quite normal sequel of childbirth.

Nowadays, at home, when the woman thinks she may be in labour, apart from seeing that everything is ready and the baby's clothes are aired, she continues with her normal daily routine until she feels that the moment has arrived when she wants to concentrate upon her labour. By this time she is probably already half dilated, and the apparent length of her labour has been noticeably shortened simply because she has been up and about and her mind has been occupied. (In some big hospitals there are sitting-rooms where the mother can wait and watch television during the early part of the first stage, but these are the exception rather than the rule.) She goes to her familiar room surrounded by the furniture, books, and pictures she likes. Her husband has returned from work to be with her and they sit quietly together, chatting between contractions, and, when they are big enough to need coping with, working together to achieve a harmonious reaction to them in the way that is described in Chapter 8. The midwife, often a friend already, looks in to see that everything is all right and tells them how far the cervix is dilated. They listen to the baby's heart-beats through the stethoscope and are very thrilled. She may go away again, promising to look in later, and leaving her telephone number so that they can get her quickly. Some time later husband and wife realize that they are approaching

1. Free movement rather than the immobilization of the abdominal muscles is the quickest way to get one's figure back.

2. Drinking much more than one wants is more likely to diminish rather than to increase the milk supply. Women are naturally thirsty when nursing, but there is no need for them to drink more than they wish. Water, milk, cocoa, malt drinks, fruit juices, beer – even champagne – are all suitable.

the end of the first stage; he has made drinks for her and fetched ice from the fridge to refresh and cool her and has rung up the midwife to tell her that things are really moving. She arrives in time to help the mother through the difficult transition phase, whilst the husband assists them both. They form a team working harmoniously towards the same end. There is little need for talk, as each understands what the other is trying to do. The room is very peaceful; there is only the sound of the mother's careful rhythmic breathing and an occasional word of encouragement or advice from the husband or midwife.

The mother is cold, and her husband brings extra blankets and a hot-water bottle and helps her to shift to a more comfortable position to ease the backache as her baby's head presses lower. Perhaps she loses the rhythm of her breathing a moment, but then her husband breathes with her so that the breathing remains light and on top of the contractions.

At last the mother feels she must push and, with her husband's arm around her, she starts pressing the baby gently but firmly down the birth canal. Soon the baby's head is visible, even before she realizes that the birth is so near. Her husband sees it first and his eyes are shining with excitement and joy as he tells her. Then she too looks down with the next contraction. Before long the whole body slides out. The mother holds the baby immediately, and after the midwife has bathed and dressed him, he is tucked up close to her, so that she can reach him, while the midwife clears up, and the husband boils the kettle for tea.

The husband and wife are left with their baby, alone in the quiet house, sharing an indescribable sense of wonder. There is an almost honeymoon atmosphere about those first days after the baby has come. The midwife comes in each day to bath the baby, unless the mother wishes to, to take the mother's temperature and pulse, and to give any help with feeding the baby that may be required.

In the familiar surroundings of home the mother is relaxed. She sleeps well, adapts herself to the baby's rhythm rather than to that imposed by hospital routine, and gradually gets to know her child and to plan her day and her other activities to fit in with her responsibilities as a mother. There is no sudden break, as when a woman comes out of hospital and tries to cope with housework and a baby whom she has hardly handled at all up to that time.

Details of how to prepare for a home confinement are given on page 263.

THE DISPLACED SIBLING

If there are already other children in the family, the introduction of the new brother or sister is made much more naturally immediately after the birth, at home, than days after when the mother has returned from hospital.[1] The toddler is allowed to touch the new baby and to 'help' with his bath. This is much better than dolls! The process of birth itself is also accepted more naturally, and is not thought of as an illness for which the mother has to be rushed to hospital. Since many babies are born at night, there may be no separation from the mother involved at all, the toddler being tucked up in bed before the mother starts her labour in earnest. This not only affects the acceptance of the new baby by the toddler, but the continuing loving relationship between the toddler and his mother, which is not suddenly threatened by her withdrawal at a moment of family crisis, the excitement of which the small child must sense.

The child can be brought in to see his mother and the baby as soon as the afterbirth has been delivered and put out of sight. (As he has not witnessed the birth itself, he should not see the least aesthetic aspect of it. If the afterbirth is all he sees of the birth he may think there has been some sort of butchery – and this, incidentally, holds good for the husband too.) The baby should be in his cot and not in his mother's arms when he sees him for the first time, and the mother should avoid any elaborate displays of affection for the new baby. She can point out the tiny nails and eyelashes and how little and helpless the

1. In the last few years some progressive maternity departments have started allowing other children of the family to visit. The rate of infection has not, in fact, increased as a result.

baby is – which will almost certainly invoke a response of tenderness on the part of the older child – but she should allow the first expressions of joy in the baby's birth to come from the child himself. If a doll or some other special present is waiting to celebrate the birthday the advent of the baby is made even more welcome. The toddler can sit on the bed and can be cuddled at the same time as the baby, and if a special store of biscuits or fruit is kept by the mother's bed for feeding times, and toys and other materials for quiet occupations are in her room, they can be very pleasant and looked forward to rather than resented by the displaced child. By no word or action should the mother suggest that the older child intends to hurt the baby, and he should instead be given positive encouragement and help to hold him correctly.

When grandparents, relations and other visitors arrive, a toddler who enjoys it can be the person who takes them to the new baby and shows him to them. In this way the new baby belongs to him too and is not simply a rival.

All these things are difficult or impossible to organize in hospital, and the resulting jealousy is likely to be more acute, painful for the toddler and difficult for the mother to cope with in the early weeks after the baby's birth, when she least wants to be troubled with psychological problems of this kind, and has the least time to deal with them.

But however well the parents have organized the birth and the care of the toddler, and however careful they have been to give him plenty of attention and to make him feel loved and wanted, they should not resent him or feel that they have a maladjusted child, or that they are hopeless failures as parents, if the toddler shows overt or concealed jealousy later, perhaps when the baby is beginning to acquire new skills and is the object of much adult attention as he takes his first steps or says his first words. Some parents feel that in having done all they could to counteract jealousy it should not make its appearance at all, and some forget that it is not only or even mainly in the early weeks that the jealousy may be most apparent, but that it may become noticeable after the novelty of the baby has worn off. Sibling jealousy is a perfectly natural phenomenon and one that parents must expect to confront however skilled their management of the toddler. Whilst removing the baby from danger, it is important for the parents to face up to any shock or horror they may feel at the signs of jealousy they observe in their toddlers; shock is a most unhelpful emotion and inhibits positive action. Home confinement does not eliminate sibling jealousy, but it can defer its appearance and possibly also lessen its intensity.

To conclude: the birth of a child is a *family* event and as such should, ideally, take place at home as a normal part of life. If there are clinical contra-indications, or if it is a first baby, a 48-hour bed can be booked, but if everything is likely to be straightforward home may be the best place. We have in Britain a district midwifery system of which we can be very proud, and local midwives are usually highly skilled women dedicated to their calling.

CHAPTER 3

The Psychology of Pregnancy

HERE we are concerned not with the physical development of the foetus and the birth of the baby, but with some feelings about having a baby which any single individual may or may not have but which are sufficiently common to require some sort of description.

SOME EMOTIONAL STATES COMMON TO PREGNANCY

We hear a great deal about the increased sensitivity and emotionalism of the pregnant woman. By tradition she is unstable, unpredictable, easily driven to tears, with strange, illogical desires and fancies. She is the essence of irrational femininity.

Why does she behave like this? What are her longings and her secret fears? From what is she trying to escape?

The mother who is preparing herself for childbirth by reading and by learning the techniques which may enable her to enjoy a natural birth is less likely to suffer from the extremes of emotional unpredictability than the woman who faces birth ignorant and fearful. But, however knowledgeable a woman and however great her trust in herself, she tends to be more vulnerable than usual – more quickly disgusted and nauseated by the ugly and the cruel, more readily thrilled by beauty and tenderness. As Christmas comes, to give but one instance, the image of the Child in the manger is for her not the sentimental symbol which it may have been up till then, but brings with it the wonder of the promise of new life. She is peculiarly receptive and unusually sensitive.

There is an emotional rationale in the behaviour of the pregnant woman and its nature repays some examination. The basis of this apparent unreasonableness lies in a psychological logic, the structure of which I shall attempt to trace in the following pages.

Inability to adjust to the role of pregnancy and motherhood

However much they dreamed of having a baby the realization that they have conceived comes to many women as a shock, and often as one not wholly pleasant, especially when the child is conceived within a few months of marriage and when the husband and wife are still taking the first steps in learning to live together. Suddenly the girl is somebody different – an expectant mother – a subject of interest and concern to society; her life seems to be no longer intimate and apart, but something anybody can talk about. They even know when her last period was, whether she is being sick in the morning, and whether her nipples are the 'right' shape. She goes to the hospital where her urine and blood are tested, her blood pressure is taken and she is sounded with stethoscopes and patted and tapped. This is all, to say the least, a sudden, if necessary, invasion of privacy.

Sometimes it is made still more of a shock for the woman by the nature of the organization of the clinic. She has to sit around with a great many other expectant mothers for anything up to three or four hours in a gloomy and sometimes obviously dirty waiting-room where they are all discussing their insides. The conversation is aggressively feminine and anti-male. She is ushered from one herd to the next, outside cubicles where she is told to undress and don a white smock; the smell of stale sweat sickens and disgusts her and she waits shivering with apprehension. At last the door is flung open and a nurse helps her to lie on a hard, high table to be examined by an impersonal doctor who may not bother to say good afternoon, who prods and pushes and presses his hand painfully into her groin, finally sliding his fingers into her vagina. He rarely tells her that everything is all right, but looks grave and preoccupied and leaves her to imagine the worst. He may not tell her that the baby is lying in a good position, or allow her to listen to the quick, powerful heart-beats, which would reassure her enormously. Before she has had time to ask a single question she is told to get down and informed that she must come again in four weeks' or two weeks' or a week's time.

Perhaps it was only a few months ago that this girl was married, in orange blossom and white, followed by the thrill of the honeymoon. Only months before that perhaps she had first been kissed by the man and had felt her body responding with physical excitement. It was all romantic and gay, and she wondered if it would finish as in the fairy tales ' . . . and so they married, and lived happily ever after.'

Suddenly the romance and the dream are shattered. A baby is on the way. She is no longer a girl, like the others in the office; something has set her apart from them now. A new life is growing inside her. Joking remarks are made and everyone is interested in her 'condition'. Many girls who are unprepared for this transition find themselves confronted with a role – that of the expectant mother – which they are unable or unwilling to play. They are emotionally unprepared for motherhood and the fact that they are pregnant, and sometimes hate themselves for it. The role of mother was previously seen only in others; but now the girl is called upon, relentlessly forced by the growing child inside her, to act a part she does not know, a part at once unfamiliar and frightening.

She may first of all try to disguise her pregnancy as far as possible. She chooses her clothes carefully so as to hide the fact of her thickening waist; she may see herself as much slimmer than she is and go through the whole or most of her pregnancy believing that 'it does not show'. She irritates her husband with her constant question, 'You wouldn't think I was pregnant, would you?' and remarks about other women who seem to her to look much more pregnant than she does.

Her main concern at first is in not losing her figure too soon and in getting it back again immediately after the birth – not unworthy aims in themselves, but sometimes symptomatic of a deeper disturbance associated with a denial of her role as mother.

A woman's difficulty in adjusting to the role of pregnancy

and motherhood is increased by a general lack of clarity in masculine and feminine roles within our society at this time. The woman does not know what she is supposed to be or how she should 'see' herself. She is perfectly aware that her role must be different from that of her grandmother – and from that of her mother. But she finds it difficult to form an ideal image of herself as a person with her own ideas and achievements, which nevertheless allows her the satisfactions deriving from full acceptance of the roles of wife and mother.

The educated, middle-class woman is supposed to be all things to a man; she is to turn herself into a many-coloured kaleidoscope of personalities and to become cook, courtesan, intellectual comrade, sympathetic mother, gay mistress, tender first love, help-meet in man's trials, and social hostess. She goes out to work, bakes his bread, rears his children, makes his curtains, does a little oil painting in her spare time. A woman cannot open a magazine without reading of achievements in *haute cuisine*, beauty culture, interior decoration, woodwork, plumbing, how to get on with the boss and how to look attractive at 8 p.m. after having been in the office all day in the same clothes.

This suggests a general lack of acceptance of the roles of wife and mother as they have been known for centuries in Western society. They are no longer sufficient, and increasing demands are being made upon women. Essentially they are required to take on all men's tasks and characteristics without relinquishing any of their femininity and charm.

Under these circumstances, unless a woman is capable of very drastic and rapid adjustments in her daily life, pregnancy and motherhood may be a strain for her. She struggles hard to avoid getting bogged down in domestic routine, but when she becomes pregnant and she becomes aware of the limitations of her activities in pregnancy, and later, of the bondage of small children, she sometimes begins to feel trapped by forces now right outside her own control.

Society is interested in and concerned about her – not for herself and her achievements, but only because she is the bearer of new life. She does not matter. The baby does. She is

warned to look after herself, to get sufficient rest, to eat
nourishing food, not to go in aeroplanes, on boats, and in fast
cars, and she resents feeling herself merely a vessel for the baby.
Mothers-in-law can be particularly irritating in this respect.
Sometimes she longs to do something shocking – to ski,
dance all night or have a love affair, thereby cocking a snook
at society and its dictates.

When couples have been married only a short time and did
not expect that the wife would conceive so soon, interpersonal
problems which could have been slowly worked out through
the months of early marriage may come to a head. If the wife is
suffering from severe pregnancy nausea and her breasts are
swollen and aching, and if she feels that all her physical at-
tractions are being swept away by unwelcome maternity,
intercourse can no longer be the ritual by which quarrels are
patched up and by which physical closeness takes the place of
a lack of understanding between two people who may be finding it hard to adjust to each other. However, some women who
feel that they 'should' desire their husbands force themselves
to make love, but are unable to experience orgasm, which
may lead to unresolved feelings of guilt (nowadays the effect
of sex education has been such that women think they 'ought'
to reach physical orgasm at each act of intercourse).

The woman may no longer be able to make love with the
same unselfconscious abandon, and this is further complicated
by the fact that she feels that her husband cannot continue to
desire her with a body spreading in all directions like this, and
she is afraid of losing his love. She is acutely aware of each
honeymoon tenderness forgotten, each little gesture of love
and intimacy neglected. She may weep all morning over the
kiss he forgot to give her. She needs his demonstrated affection for her as never before. Unless her husband makes a
deliberate effort to share with her in preparations for the birth
and to become interested in the details of the unknown experience that lies before her, she may feel very alone and unwanted. She feels as if, in the words of one mother, 'we are
not going along the same path any longer', or, as another said,
'I feel I'm growing farther and farther away from him.'

Some women suffer the strain of never being able to talk to their husband about their pregnancy, their confinement, or the new baby, because the husband seems to close his mind to it all, ignores the fact that his wife is pregnant, as far as possible, and tries to act as if it were nothing to do with him anyway and it is all 'a woman's affair'. To such women pregnancy, in spite of wanting the baby, can be a really unhappy time.

With a few women it is much worse. To them childbirth is even a threat. They feel physically nauseated by the body of the child developing within them like a parasite, drawing life from them. They feel horrified by the inevitability of the process once it has started, horrified at the thickening of their bodies and at the movements of the kicking baby. But even here the husband's attitude and loving care may be able to affect the woman's adjustment, and if he is able to accept the whole process as natural and to let her know that she still has his love she may be better able to accept her pregnancy instead of fighting it.

The need for information and reassurance

But whether or not a woman wants a child, whether or not she enjoys the state of pregnancy as such, and whatever the treatment she receives from her husband, her relationship with her doctor and midwife, or with the hospital or clinic staff, must enter into the reckoning and affect the way in which she approaches her labour.

The expectant mother is particularly sensitive to any suggestion that things may not be quite as they should be. She stores in her mind each word uttered by the obstetrician when he examines her. Since these tend to be few and far between it is not difficult to remember what he said and to go home to brood over their exact significance. 'We ought to keep an eye on you. . . .' Why? Something must be wrong! 'We must check your blood pressure each week from now on. . . .' Am I developing toxaemia . . .? District midwives talk much more to their patients as a rule, and spend some time in explaining matters and in making sure that the mother understands.

Women need to become familiar with certain common medical terms simply in order to understand what their doctor and midwife are talking about, since it can be very distressing for a patient to hear a conversation about her inside in purely technical terms which she cannot understand, and she often thinks they mean much worse than in fact they do. Every intelligent woman has a right to know what the doctors and nurses are talking about in front of her and to have the difficulties explained, if there are any. Usually, however, there are no difficulties and technical parlance serves merely to create a screen between attendants and patient, a screen which makes her feel that they have something they want to hide from her. This is not the sort of situation that allays fear and creates a confident attitude in the woman.

It is important also that the obstetrician should take the little extra time needed to tell her that her baby is fine and that everything is going ahead splendidly. This would provide her with an emotional cocktail instead of the sense of depression she so often has as she emerges from the clinic or hospital. More than one woman has cried herself to sleep after attending a clinic which has left her feeling an anonymous 'case'. If the husband can arrange to go with his wife to the clinic, even though he may be the only man there, it will give her great moral support. Wherever possible the husband should meet the obstetrician or midwife and help his wife talk over arrangements for the kind of birth she wants.

There are still obstetricians and nurses who need to be far more aware of the impression they create upon their patients. Some would be appalled if they realized what they thought about them. I know that one obstetrician who prides himself upon his sympathy is described by more than one patient as 'unapproachable' and 'always so rushed'. His skill does not extend to any deep understanding of his relationship with his patients. This is partly due to lack of time. He cannot be bothered with inessentials and with the niceties of polite conversation when so much that is urgent is waiting to be done. But it is partly due also to a tradition that there must exist a social distance between doctor and patient, which serves to maintain his dignity and status *vis-à-vis* the layman and to make his pronouncements worthy of respect. The 'bedside manner' disappeared with the doctor who acted the part of kindly father-confessor and avuncular adviser – a role which itself served to maintain this distance by its assumption of implicit authority and superior status – and in his place has come the clinician, the foreman and manager of the baby factory, who treats the women lying on the examination tables as if they were so many fish on a slab. The only way in which this can be altered is for women, and their husbands, to protest politely.

It is not only the woman who is obviously disturbed who may need help. A woman may be doing fine and taking pregnancy in her stride – asserting, as she downs her third whisky or smokes the twentieth cigarette that 'it doesn't make any difference to me'. She may confront labour with an over-brisk cheerfulness: 'It's just like shelling peas', or refuse antenatal preparation and react violently against a concentration of ideas on motherhood and the coming baby with, 'I'm sick and tired of all the talk', or 'Hens don't make all that fuss' (some do).

Straightforward fear of childbirth is not the commonly confronted obstacle that once it was, and giving accurate information may be all that is required to dispel it. After all, it is safer nowadays to have a baby than to drive in Bank Holiday traffic. But it often comes disguised under a cloak of apparent nonchalance and sometimes is symptomatic of a deeper anxiety, where the woman feels humiliated or trapped by her pregnancy, or confronts problems which make her particularly liable to depression during, or more often after, her pregnancy. Unless it is plain that she is severely disturbed it still happens too often that everyone tries to jolly her out of it: 'It's just glands' and (to her husband): 'Take her to the pictures' – which is about as much use as the often recommended glass of wine at bed-time for the frigid wife.

Unless and until doctors have the time and skill to interest themselves in the psychological care of pregnant women there will remain a vast field of therapy which is at the moment largely left to chance and haphazard concern. David Stafford-

Clark[1] points out that if 'the actual proportion of time in the medical curriculum devoted to the teaching of psychiatry ... were to approach in proportion the size of the problem which the qualified doctor must meet in his practice, a great deal of the existing balance and emphasis in medical training and in medical examinations would have to be changed.' Similarly midwives, who might find it easier to get closer than the busy general practitioner to their patients and to understand what was going on in their minds, are also hampered by lack of training in psychology except of a very rudimentary kind, and of course they too are often grossly overworked.

Depression a month before confinement

Towards the end of pregnancy a great many women suffer unaccountable depression which passes off as suddenly as it came and for no apparent reason. I have noticed that among women attending my classes there is a time between the sixth and the third week before the expected date of confinement when their self-confidence is at its lowest, when childhood fears become dominant, and when they become most impatient with pregnancy. The fact that a woman knows that this 'stage fright' is normal and that many other women pass through it should help her tolerate it. Extravagant as it may be, a new kaftan, a cape or ear-rings, or any other buy kept until this time will help lift morale. It is important to get out and to enjoy some entertainment and recreation, and whilst rest is necessary, if the mother can arrange something to look forward to each day her thoughts will cease to centre only on her pregnancy and the weight inside her. In my experience this depression prior to the birth is a mental state to be foreseen, and is indeed much more common than the depression which follows childbirth on or about the third day after, which one hears so much about.

1. David Stafford-Clark, *Psychiatry To-day*, Penguin Books, 1951.

Wanting to kick over the traces

It is as well to begin regular practising of this method as early in pregnancy as possible, any time after the third month. However, this book is full of 'shoulds' and 'oughts', and any woman who does not make a fetish of training herself for childbirth is bound to want to rebel against the self-imposed discipline and kick over the traces occasionally, to feel gay, free and undisciplined, to forget that she is pregnant, to eat and drink what she likes, to forget her exercises.

This is completely healthy and admirable behaviour. To allow for an occasional week or so when preparation is neglected, therefore, it is important to start early. One can then proceed in a leisurely fashion, not being driven on by lack of time and the urgency of getting in the instruction before labour takes one unawares.

Fear that the baby will be malformed

Any time after about the fifth month of pregnancy when the child begins to move and becomes a reality to the mother, she may start to think about her baby as possibly deformed. Especially if she has taken any drugs the effects of which she does not know in early pregnancy, she may think back to the 'thalidomide babies'. This fear may be recognized consciously, or be presented in the unconscious life of the dream and but rarely brought to full consciousness. It is a very real terror. What if this thing I am nourishing and cherishing within my own body, around which my whole life is built now, whose pulse beats fast deep within me – what if this child should prove to be a hideous deformed creature, sub-human, a thing I should be able to love, but which I would shudder to see?

It is useless to force oneself not to brood on such things, because the more one pushes these imaginings out of one's conscious mind, the more tightly they pack the world of dreams. Every unwise remark made by midwife or doctor indicates the possibility of this happening and confirms the mother's fears. 'The baby's very small, you know....' 'Does it move much?...' Nor is it sufficient to explain that only 3 per 1,000 babies are born mentally defective, or to provide other kinds of statistical evidence for disproving the woman's fears. If 997 babies are normal, how much worse it seems for her baby to be abnormal.

This sort of fear is associated with the crystallization of deep-seated feelings of guilt. The girl wants to punish herself, to wipe away her guilt by atonement – by producing this monstrosity from within her own body, the living embodiment of her own evil. This most personal, most intimate offering to life from the core of one's own body, out from its enveloping darkness and secrecy – this is contaminated and diseased. Once this can be brought up to the conscious mind – and accepted – half the force of the terror has gone. This is not a private, individual fear. It is something shared by many pregnant women, although a few may laugh at it. Once one realizes that one is not alone in this experience one escapes from the individual-centred pain it involves. One is no longer enclosed in oneself, fighting it in darkness.

The first question of many new mothers who have gone through this fear, and who may not have come to terms with it or understood it, as their baby slips out into the world is, 'Is it all right?' At this moment they are unmasked. Their question is urgent, imperative. They are not yet aware even of the baby as a person – but only as their own offering, squirming out of the darkness – 'Is it all right?' They must see the baby immediately to know for themselves the truth, must hold it and see its perfection and wholeness. No wonder that they laugh and cry at the same time. Unless the deformity in a baby is very severe, the mother should always see it at once. Sugar-loaf moulding of a persistent occipito-posterior (the baby who is born face to pubis) which results in a temporarily very high-domed head, the peculiar shape of head of a baby who has been presenting by the face – pressure marks (little pink blotches often on the baby's eyelids and between the eyes), marks of the forceps, haematoma, which is a temporary swelling a bit like a large blister on the baby's head – the result of pressure on the soft tissues, and not in any way affecting the baby's brain – these are all easily explained, and should be explained, by the doctor or midwife, but when a mother does not see her baby she imagines much worse things. Indeed in the interval between the baby's birth and the time when she is actually permitted to see him she may be so sure that something is wrong with the child that reassurance may come with great difficulty, even when the child is peacefully sucking in her arms and it is to all intents and purposes a normal, healthy baby.

SOME OTHER PROBLEMS OF PREGNANCY

I have found that women who suffer from chronic constipation are likely to doubt their ability to give birth spontaneously (they just do not believe in the smooth functioning of their bodies). Frequently, but by no means always, this is linked with sexual maladjustment. They need to learn to adjust themselves to a natural and *internal* rhythm, whether it be that of defecation, of orgasm, or of labour contractions. The constipated woman needs help, not only because straining is bad for her both during pregnancy and post-natally, but because a basic mistrust of her physiological processes may be a threat to her equilibrium in labour.

Whether or not the constipation is of psychological origin – and there are obviously all sorts of physiological and dietary reasons why a woman may be constipated – the very fact that she has lost faith in the ability of her body to work smoothly and easily may make her very likely to distrust its efficiency in childbearing.

Apart from obvious remedies of diet, there are three approaches to smooth bowel functioning. Firstly, her developing body awareness, which comes with training in progressive and differential relaxation, will help her to observe more carefully and accurately exactly how her body works in defecation. Secondly, her ability to contract and relax the muscles of the pelvic floor at will, which she learns through pelvic floor exercises, will allow her to release the *levator ani* during the act of defecation. Thirdly, practice in gentle, smooth bearing down in a rounded-back and bent-knee position will help her to adopt a good posture for defecation, and to press from above downwards, rather than resisting the natural process by squeezing up from below and using unnatural force in order to get rid of the faeces. She should practise unstrained bearing down during defecation, and will notice that in the bowel rhythm there is a right moment and a wrong moment to bear down; if she allows herself gradually to feel the right moment at which to do this, it is in itself not only a valuable preparation for labour but builds up trust in her body.

Constipation is just one example. An allied problem is that of the woman who compulsively desires to rid herself of whatever has entered into her (child, faeces or penis) whether it be expressed in the form of *hyperemesis gravidarum* (repeated and constant cyclical vomiting of pregnancy), which in severe cases can last right through the pregnancy and make the woman very ill indeed, habitual spontaneous abortion of psychological origin, or over-vigorous and insensitive efforts to expel the foetus in the second stage of labour. Emphasis on the need to expel the child rapidly and to make the best use of one's powers (and the use by the antenatal teacher of the aggressively military imagery favoured by some English exponents of psychoprophylaxis) may in such cases reinforce and give positive sanction to this compulsive striving in labour. This not only adds to the stress and turmoil of the second stage, but the experience of childbirth itself can thereby even be incorporated into the pattern of mental illness.

THE WOMAN WHO HAS FOUND IT DIFFICULT TO CONCEIVE

There are special problems too for the woman who has been trying to start a baby for a long time, who has attended fertility clinics and been through the mill of all the tests and examinations, and for whom sexual intercourse has become a means of trying to conceive a child rather than something enjoyable in itself. If this continues for any length of time a man can feel humiliated and unloved, and this in turn must affect the quality of marriage. Sometimes a woman uses a man rather like a queen bee the drone – merely to fertilize her. Perhaps she pleads with him to make love although he is tired, not because she really wants him, but because her temperature chart has indicated that this is about the time of ovulation. As soon as she misses her first period she then has nothing more to do with him, intent on protecting the nascent life within her. It is understandable that the man may be resentful and may feel that he has been used like a stud bull.

Moreover the woman herself may have little confidence in her ability to bear a child and be beset with fears that the baby will be abnormal, or that she will lose it during pregnancy. She may also have become highly dependent on hospital staff, feeling that if she needed help with conceiving it, how much more is she likely to need assistance with bearing the child. Women who are going through this sort of stress benefit greatly from belonging to a class where they have an opportunity to talk to and share experiences with other expectant mothers. Far from not making love in case it is a threat to the pregnancy, I find these women relax better if explicit approval is given to lovemaking, except for times when the period would have been due during the first months, and since it is sometimes their own tension which is the greatest risk to the pregnancy, this can only be to the good. In fact, a parallel can be drawn between the deep psychophysical release after orgasm and the complete relaxation of mind and body needed in labour.

THE HUSBAND'S JEALOUSY OF THE UNBORN CHILD

Some women become so wrapped up in their pregnancies with their minds centred around their navels that their husbands become quite miserable and feel very lonely and unwanted. Even a wife who thinks she is doing everything reasonable to let her husband know that she still loves him may find that he resents her pregnancy and feels unloved in much the same way as he may once have done before when his mother presented him with a baby brother or sister. He feels cast out in a similar fashion and is secretly jealous of the baby.

If this happens a woman should realize that it is probably no reflection on her abilities as a wife. He is simply expressing the tensions, frustration and loneliness that he felt as a child in relation to younger siblings. She should take especial care to show her continuing love for him, and not hesitate to demonstrate her affection. He wants to feel needed, and the preparations for the baby should take him into account too.

Living, as he did, within a patriarchal society which has now been superseded, Freud described a culture in which women envied men for all that they possessed, the symbol of much of this jealousy being crystallized in penis envy, but men envied women not at all, since they were inferior beings anyway. Ian Suttie suggested, however, that men might envy women their power of bearing children, and believed that the practice of the 'couvade' known in many primitive societies, whereby the husband is treated as if he and not his wife were having the baby, and goes into labour instead of her, was 'an expression of unconscious desire on the part of the husband to share in the production of the child'.[1] This jealousy which differs from the previous type in that it is jealousy not of the new baby but of the woman's ability to be with child, Suttie calls 'Zeus jealousy', since Zeus swallowed his pregnant wife in order to bear her child himself.

It seems to me that there are several patterns of this jealousy which we can trace during a woman's pregnancy. Some men are aware of it consciously. As the wife becomes more engrossed with her pregnancy, with the fascinating movements of the child within her and her dreams of what the child will be like, the husband, as we have seen, may feel more and more shut out. An experience which is obviously of vital and fundamental importance in his wife's life is denied him. The wife, unaware of her husband's isolation, interprets his questions and his concern for her, by which he expresses his desire to enter into her world, as fussiness and may scorn his care and over-protectiveness. Or he may withdraw into a man's

1. Ian Suttie, *Origins of Love and Hate*, Kegan Paul, 1935.

world, asserting his masculine role aggressively and pretend to take no interest in his wife's condition or in her hopes or fears about labour. Then she very soon becomes deeply hurt.

It is significant that couples who prepare together for labour and who share the experience of childbirth are far less likely to have this feeling of separation from each other during pregnancy, and the husband is less liable to feel abandoned and alone in this way. He feels that the child is his child as much as his wife's and that he too has helped to make it, not only in the sense that he scattered sperm and started the growth of the foetus in a split moment of time, but in the sense that he is in a much deeper and wider sense the child's creator. In accepting the full responsibility of paternity he is rewarded with a sense of achievement, and indeed, some husbands find it difficult to imagine how their wives could have a successful pregnancy and labour without them, just as many wives find the idea of labour without their husband's presence a very unpleasant prospect and one which, given the choice, they would not willingly endure.

SEX IN PREGNANCY

Most of the books on sex in marriage and on marriage guidance neglect the very important subject of sex in pregnancy and after the baby comes, and of the developing relationship between husband and wife as they together create a child. If we are to consider not only a woman's body, but the woman as a person, and not merely the experience through which she is passing, but that experience in the context of the life of the growing family, it is necessary to say something about the husband and wife relationship in the physical sense.

However, this is by no means the whole of a woman's sexuality. Intercourse is only one aspect of it, and menstruation, pregnancy, birth and breast-feeding are all part of the totality which comprises her sexual role. There is, for instance, an ebb and flow in a woman's desire for intercourse which closely corresponds to these other functions, and these are not isolated each from the other, but are interdependent parts of her sexual cycle.

The taboo on intercourse during all or part of pregnancy and in the immediate post-natal period varies enormously between different societies and even within societies, as between different social classes for instance. What women *feel* about this is probably just as important as straight medical fact, and if a woman finds intercourse distasteful in late pregnancy, or during menstruation, persuading her that she should be able to take a more rational view, and that this taboo is just a remnant of dark myths rooted in pre-history, is not only unlikely to be very successful but may do positive harm.

Intercourse can continue throughout pregnancy, with the emphasis upon a careful tenderness. Great unhappiness is caused some wives by their husband's refusal to make love, and some husbands also hate their wives' pregnancies because they think they are prohibited not only intercourse but all love play. In a normal marriage between two healthy individuals the husband is not a threat to his wife at this time; she wants him and needs him as at any other time. One woman spoke to me of the distress she felt at her husband's refusal to make love because he had read in a book that during the first three months of pregnancy, the three months preceding childbirth and the three months after it, a couple should not have intercourse. She said they were both unhappy about this and her husband was feeling very frustrated. He thought that if he allowed himself to penetrate her 'the bag of waters would burst' and premature labour would immediately result. Many couples have proved that this is nonsense.

If the woman has previously miscarried it is wise to avoid actual intercourse when the second and third periods are due. Only if there is bleeding during the present pregnancy need intercourse be avoided till after the third period has been missed. But it is not, of course, necessary to deny the husband all sexual pleasure and the ejaculation can take place outside the woman's body.

Forgoing complete intercourse if there is risk of miscarriage may be as important for the woman *psychologically* as for any other reason. She should be able to feel that she has guarded the foetus so far as lies in her power, and can feel terribly guilty when she has a miscarriage. So often women rack their brains as they lie immobilized and bleeding, feeling utterly miserable, and wondering whether it was that second martini last Tuesday, or running for the bus, or getting worked up about mother-in-law coming to stay. Often each additional miscarriage contributes to a woman's conviction that she is an utter failure, and this must have an effect in the long run not only on her child-bearing but on her marriage.

As the woman becomes larger it is necessary to devise new positions so that she can be comfortable, and at no time should the man's whole weight rest upon her, or great pressure be put upon the uterus, either from outside or from the conventional position in which the man lies full length on top of the woman with the force of the penis against the cervix. Indeed, this is a very poor one for pregnancy, and also for afterwards, when the wife's breasts may be very full and tender. The use of extra pillows can add greatly to comfort and pleasure.

A few women dislike intercourse throughout pregnancy. They feel they have become, as it were, sacred vessels of new life and thus should not be 'contaminated' by sex. But to many women the upsurge of happiness that comes with the realization of pregnancy brings with it intense delight in the sexual relationship – if not immediately, at least after the difficult first few months when any nausea is over.

Many women go through a period during a pregnancy when they do not seem able to 'give' both to a man and to the baby inside them – and of course the same feeling can exist during the puerperium, when it can be a cause of real marital tension. A woman is more likely to be sexually unresponsive if her husband has made derisive comments about her changing figure, so he bears part responsibility for this. But if a woman should find herself turning inward in this way, lying in bed waiting for the next bump from within the uterus rather than being able luxuriously to enjoy her husband's love-making, it might be as well for her to use additional aids to get herself more into the romantic mood. (Every woman knows what they are: scent, wine, soft music, frilly lingerie, flattering lighting; it is not only her husband who will react to the right mood – she will find herself entering better into the spirit of the thing.)

Sheer tiredness can, of course, be a cause of the relative frigidity that crops up in pregnancy (and after childbirth). Sometimes during pregnancy a couple of days away together in a hotel solves the problem, or even a whole day in bed (alone) with the glossies. If neither of these can be managed a woman can try to get a sleep sometime during the day, so that she is fresh and attractive for him. It is as much a question of breaking the old routine, of doing something new and of getting out of the rut as of getting a few more hours in which to sleep; habitually lying in bed in the morning with toast crumbs between the sheets and marmalade sticking to the bedside table does not do a thing to help, and just makes a woman feel more wretched.

Some women dislike intercourse towards the end of pregnancy and some fear that it may harm the baby. After the baby has dropped into the pelvis it feels as if there is very little space left. If one thinks how very painful a full bladder can be to a woman in the last weeks of pregnancy, one will realize that the erect penis can also cause pain unless it is inserted very gently. Even then it may make the wife uncomfortable if it is introduced deeply, and it is wiser to introduce only the tip.

Some women get strong uterine contractions when they make love. This occurs during the woman's orgasm. Each woman will know perfectly well herself if this is so with her. Nearly always they will die down and disappear altogether if she lies quietly, perhaps with a hot water bottle against her abdomen or in the small of her back to help her relax – although that is not very difficult to achieve after making love. Occasionally, however, labour might be initiated. But this is only likely to happen when she is ripe for labour anyway. Many couples have used this as a way of inducing labour which everyone was ready and waiting for. In some societies intercourse just before the onset and during the early first stage of labour is thought to be highly efficacious and to ensure a speedy and safe birth. This is often explained by informants in terms of lubricating the birth canal, and it was believed in the North of England until quite recently. But since, because the upper segment of the uterus is contracting, violent orgasm on the part of the woman can trigger off premature labour in this way, during the last two or three weeks many couples prefer to enjoy gentler forms of satisfaction. If a woman does not mentally commit herself to the idea of physical orgasm, or at least to a very tumultuous one, she can still feel in harmony with her husband's joy and a pleasure gained through sympathy and love. A couple can take pregnancy as an opportunity to explore other methods of erotic satisfaction. Intercourse itself is an excellent exercise for the muscles of the pelvic floor, and if a woman finds complete relaxation difficult in her preparation for childbirth she should note the full neuro-muscular release that comes after orgasm. That is evidence of her ability to relax.

I believe that both man and woman should aim at mutuality and equal caring rather than exploitation of the marriage relationship. Yet every man wants to see his wife as a harlot occasionally. A woman should not always wait for the initiation of sex play, but should study how best she can seduce her husband. It is a pity if pregnancy causes them to lose the gaiety of early married life. Sometimes as we have seen a man fears that the baby is in some way his rival. He needs to be reassured that he is not only loved, and loved deeply, but also desired passionately, and that this sort of feeling is quite different from the tenderness a woman feels for the baby inside her.

MOTHERS AND DAUGHTERS: A SECTION FOR HUSBANDS AND WIVES TO CONSIDER TOGETHER

The girl who is over-dependent upon her mother may run into severe emotional problems in childbirth and afterwards. There is even a special name for her, invented by two Swiss psychologists, de Senarclens and Picot – 'the infantile *primipara*'.[1]

This is really nothing to do with chronological age – although girls in their teens and women having their first babies are most likely to fall into this category. It is much more a matter of the degree of emotional maturity – how far the girl is able and willing to stand on her own feet, tackle her own problems and live her own life, rather than whether she is in her teens or twenties.

A girl who is still clinging to her mother in infantile dependence – and in whose marriage her mother is dominant and really the main power figure in an emotional triangle – is likely to find labour a shattering experience. During pregnancy if she goes to classes in preparation for childbirth she tends to lean on the teacher – just as she later does on her midwife – more or less helpless and passive, drinking it all in like a sponge, dutifully following prescribed mechanical techniques, obeying instructions implicitly, and trusting the teacher rather than her own body. Many teachers make the mistake of thinking her an easy pupil, who is pretty well bound to have a straightforward and happy labour. But it all really depends on the sort of support she gets when actually in labour; if she gets good support, results in terms of 'performance' are often excellent. But there is still a problem – which sooner or later will catch up with her – the basic emotional problem of over-dependence on her mother, or on other women – antenatal teachers and midwives for instance – who fit the mother image. She is launched on motherhood utterly unprepared for its responsibilities and stresses, the necessary decision-making involved in infant care, and, in urban communities, for the social isolation of the middle-class mother tied to the house and to young children. It is not surprising that many a girl like this cracks up during those early years of motherhood, becoming a dissatisfied, emotionally overwrought and unavoidably self-centred housebound wife, unable to cope with the

1. See proceedings of 1er Congrès International de Médecine Psychosomatique et Maternité, July 1962 (Société Française de Médecine Psychosomatique, rue Chanez, Paris 16e).

baby, and driving herself frantic over problems of feeding the child and of organizing the household.

Pregnancy, as we have seen, brings with it a change in social role, from bride to mother, and often from career girl to housewife, and normally an accompanying satisfying new image of the self. These are such enormous changes in identity that sometimes, almost for the first time, a girl comes face to face with what she is and what she wants to be. It is, in fact, a tremendous opportunity for growing up emotionally.

The infantile primipara, however, cannot see herself as anything else than as a daughter to her parents. In pregnancy she guards the child *in utero* a little like a doll. She may be late to recognize its movements – not until after the twentieth week – and when they occur strongly in late pregnancy may be very disturbed by them. Surprised at the child's animation and strength, she may interpret them as signs of aggression against her. But she often quite enjoys pregnancy and the amount of attention it brings, and while the baby is still *in utero*, requiring nothing of her, she maintains an emotional equilibrium. The real problems come afterwards.

After the birth she tends to be bewildered by the baby, to be unable to react 'maternally' (that is according to the cultural patterning of maternity in our society), and feels a failure at whatever she tries to do. She tries desperately to please the baby in the same way that she strives anxiously to please her mother, and when the child cries, and continues to cry, it seems to be crying 'at' her. This is the starting point of what is usually called 'mild post-natal depression'. People often think that this depression after childbirth is inevitable; it is referred to as the third or fourth day 'blues', but it often continues much longer than that. Its incidence does not find a place in clinical records, because it is expected and is considered too commonplace to be of note. (For all this, in some peasant societies it is completely unknown.) It is only when it does not seem to be getting any better, when the young mother is discovered again and again collapsed in tears over the kitchen sink, when her husband fails to improve the condition by his reiterated advice to 'snap out of it', that further advice is sought and the family doctor consulted. It is often then explained in terms of the unbalanced endocrine system.

In one sense of course all women with first babies are unprepared for the responsibilities of motherhood in our society. Girl children are given little or no preparation, except through doll play, for motherhood. And even their dolls are babies no longer, but teenagers with jutting breasts and elaborately back-combed hair styles. Girl children share very little in our modern two- or three-child family in the care of younger siblings, and it is accepted that baby-care is limited to the mother of the child, much of it taking place in privacy. It is rare to see a mother breast-feeding her child.

Women in our society are more or less insulated from baby-care until they are confronted with their own offspring. (And lessons in how to bath an immobile rubber doll do not really do much to prepare one for the nerve-racking experience of bathing one's own slippery, wriggling baby.) But many mothers quickly adapt themselves. The infantile primipara is faced with a more severe handicap, and she cannot make this transition into motherhood. The doll baby *in utero* is very different from the real child crying in its cot. It was automatically cared for and nourished in her body, but now she must do something about it to keep it alive. Although mothercraft classes may help, they do not solve her basic emotional overdependence, nor her inability to feel herself into the role of a mother. Her own mother is often ready to rush in to care for the new baby and to give advice, thus increasing her daughter's belief in her own inability to care for her child. When the baby cries she is alerted by its signals of distress but is unable to act constructively or meaningfully. She cannot identify herself with her mother and thus feed the child and soothe it, but behaves as if she were *herself* the baby needing care and love. And her self-pity can easily prove irritating and exhausting to those who most want to help her.

It is often the husband who can help most in this situation, and it is best of all if he can start during pregnancy, gradually weaning his wife away from her mother, and letting her see how much he loves and admires her in her new developing emotional maturity. He has an unenviable role, since he is standing protectively between his wife and her immediate family, and it often means that he will have to support her in ventures in independence and self-assertion that she makes contrary to her mother's advice – doing things in a different way not (let us face it) because it is necessarily a better way, but because it is vitally important that she should be able to make her own decisions, begin to act like an adult and see herself approvingly in her new role of mother.

In all this, encouragement and praise can be more effective than scathing criticism. Perhaps one should add that the husband who decides that pregnancy and birth are nothing to do with him anyway, and are a matter of feminine mystique, should not be surprised if his wife remains immature, and dependent on her parents more than on him.

HOW A MOTHER CAN HELP HER DAUGHTER DURING HER PREGNANCY

When a daughter is pregnant for the first time it is a problem for the mother to know how much advice she should give and how much she should try to enter into her daughter's life. She may be very thrilled, and usually is, about her daughter's pregnancy, and at the same time is a little anxious for her, worried that she may not be able to cope, perhaps with the pregnancy, perhaps also with the birth itself – and very probably with the new baby when it arrives.

Mothers want to share in their daughters' lives and are reminded vividly of their own early married days and the coming of their own first baby. Many daughters turn towards their mothers at this time, especially if there is a good relationship between them already. But grandmothers should try not to feel hurt when they do not, because it may simply mean that the girl has not matured enough to do this yet, but she almost certainly will later on.

Some daughters, for instance, are still working through a stage of adolescent rebellion, a perfectly natural, almost inevitable stage, but one which can be very awkward and complicated for all concerned, and one in which both parents have to have a great deal of tolerance. We normally think of this stage as finishing at about the time a girl gets married, if not before. But there are still a great many young women who are in this love-hate relationship with their mothers when they start their own families. This does not necessarily mean that a girl has cut loose from home and mother. Sometimes a girl is obviously dependent upon her mother – over-dependent – is ringing her up or writing to her every day, consults Mummy about everything; and Mummy usually isn't worried about this sort of daughter; she ought to be of course, but 'smother mothers', who never managed to cut the emotional umbilical cord, really love their daughters to behave like this and encourage their over-dependence. This sort of girl is in an infantile, pre-adolescent phase of relationship with her mother, and she has somehow to learn to grow up before she can become a mother herself.

But there is another sort of dependence, not so worrying, because it is really adolescent and not infantile dependence, where there is an intense love-hate relationship – where the girl looks as if she does not care a bit what her mother thinks and deliberately does everything in the very opposite way. But here too there is dependence upon mother's values, what the mother thinks, how the mother acts, and the girl is often quite consciously and deliberately relating her own standards and ways of doing things to those of her mother, and is going all out to do the opposite. Here too the girl is dependent upon her mother, but in a different and, although it does not look like it, perhaps a more grown-up sort of way, although I can see that it must be intensely irritating. She may seem very confident and self-assured, but she is not necessarily, and just like the other girl – the girl who is so obviously over-dependent – she too needs praise and reassurance from her mother, even though she is creating a situation in which it is very difficult for the grandmother to give it.

A girl really does need her mother when she is pregnant, and has her first baby, but not for teaching her the right methods and ways of doing things, nor for taking over the baby when it arrives while the daughter has a nice rest, but for letting her see her approval of her daughter in her new role as a mother. Basically the grandmother's task is to look for what she can praise and give her daughter the reassurance which can help her to build up her own image of herself as a mother.

Many grandmothers are not so good at this, partly because methods of child care and running a house, and the things we are aiming at in these activities – and even perhaps the partnership of a husband and wife in a marriage – are very different from what they were twenty or thirty years ago. Our mothers read Truby King. Perhaps they studied the careful guidance of the Montessori method of infant education. Their lives were, on the whole, at any rate in the middle classes, much more orderly and tidy. Our households must look pretty chaotic to them. Some grandmothers get worried when their daughters feed the baby when he cries, for instance, and fear that she is making a rod for her own back, or when she picks him up for a cuddle because he looks so delicious, and think back to their young days when they dared not move till the clock struck the hour for feeds.

But there is more to it than that. Often the maternal grandmother longs to take over the child herself and show her daughter how it is all done, to protect her (she probably sees it as that). And just when her daughter needs reassurance that her baby is perfect – (and how many mothers both during pregnancy when they can't see the child and have to take it on faith – and even later when it is born – fear that it is in some way not perfect!) – when the new mother is going through these frightening feelings of concern for the child and that she somehow cannot produce from her body something quite perfect, just then the grandmother asks worriedly, 'Do you think he's getting enough milk dear? Don't you think your milk looks rather blue and watery?' or 'He isn't very fat, is he?' or 'Shouldn't he have a tooth by now?' These things are all said with the kindest of intentions, but emphasize the grandmother's lack of confidence in her daughter as a mother just when she needs her positive support and praise.

This can be even more serious during pregnancy, when the grandmother may suggest that her daughter's actions could endanger the baby's life or mar it in some way. She must not, for example, lift her arms above her head or the cord may get tangled around the baby's neck – one well-known old wives' tale – and all this has the effect of making the girl feel more guilty.

Why should a pregnant woman feel guilty at all? Why does she not embark upon pregnancy and motherhood gaily and easily and naturally? Many girls, especially when pregnant for the first time, feel a sense of guilt, and this too in relation to their own mothers. In some way they are replacing their mothers (replacing them sexually, for pregnancy is the outward and visible sign of having had intercourse) and more than this: they are the generation which is superseding their mothers as mothers, and they often do not put this into words or even think about it, but they have the feeling that they are somehow, in some indefinable way, stealing something valuable from their mothers. It can come out into the open as a direct conflict for possession of the child, the grandmother wooing the child with sweets and presents and, the daughter says, spoiling him.

For it is not only daughters who lack confidence. Sometimes grandmothers lack confidence too. And they want to know that they are loved. They want this child to demonstrate that he loves them; and if the grandmother's own marriage is not particularly happy and she does not feel valued for her own sake, she may attempt to get this love that she needs from her daughter's children.

The future grandmother who feels unloved and unwanted can make pregnancy a particularly difficult time for her daughter.

A first pregnancy can be a time of very great stress anyway. We all know that an expectant mother is emotionally vulnerable and tends to get weepy and fly off the handle about little things, and society as a whole tolerates this with a certain degree of amusement. It is usually accounted for physiologically and put down to hormone and other changes in her body.

But this is by no means the whole of the story. There are enormous emotional adjustments to be made too, so that she can grow up enough to be not just a bride but a mother and to be able to be not only a wife to her husband but a mother to her children, and to tie these relationships together in such a way that they do not conflict.

To make this sometimes very difficult transition a girl has to be able to see herself as a mother and to like what she sees. This might be almost impossible for the girl we were talking about before, the girl in a state of adolescent rebellion, except that girls learn what it is to be a mother long before this – so a future grandmother need not worry about this. She does not need to ply her daughter with baby books and to give a lot of advice. Girls acquire these ideas most naturally and easily in childhood when they watch their mothers handling babies, whether they are their own brothers and sisters or relatives. Because they admire and love them, they see this sort of behaviour as something admirable and then start to handle their dolls or animals or baby brothers and sisters in just the same way, and to base their behaviour on their mother's. It is not really maternal instinct. It is *learned* behaviour, but learned mostly unconsciously, at an early age, when the small girl simply, naturally, as a part of her play, imitates her mother.

In cases where the mother is dead or absent and there has been an inadequate mother substitute – when the mother has been away because of illness, separation or divorce, and no one satisfactory has come to take her place, this may be absent, and then the girl has a much harder task. But even so any girl who can read and attend classes can learn all the practical details she needs to know about preparing for a baby just as she used her intelligence to learn any of the tasks she needed to know in order to hold down a job. It is a matter of getting the information and applying the intelligence.

But the thing which probably does not come so easily if there has not been a satisfactory mother in one's own childhood is the actual touch of a mother with her child, something she does not ever think about, or analyse (and probably it is better for her not to analyse it). It changes as the child gets older and is able to grow away from her a little bit and become rather more independent. The touch of a mother with a new-born child is very different from that of a mother with a nine-month-old child or a two-year-old. And the mother does not have to stop to think about it. She feels the child's needs at that time and responds appropriately. This is one of the basic things about what it is to be a good mother. All the other things – about baby baths and clothes and not sticking the safety-pin into the child – all these skills are superficial compared to that. This is one field in which self-confidence is absolutely essential, and if the girl has not got this she pauses, she *does* stop and analyse the way to do it and then she some-how cannot relate herself to the baby fully. So much that we think of as help for new mothers endangers this relationship – and makes it more difficult for the new mother to live almost as much in her baby as in herself. The almost complete pre-occupation that many new mothers feel with a new baby comes as near as possible to what it is to live in another per-son, and this is a very precious thing for the baby at this stage of its life.

The most important, the essential, help and support that any grandmother can give to her daughter is to build up this confidence in herself, a feeling of rightness about being a mother and of the way she handles her baby, and to help her relate herself to the baby. If the daughter does not seem adult, and does not seem capable of being an expert mother, there is even more reason for building up her self-confidence and giving her this sort of loving support, and thus helping her to grow up.

When a grandmother learns to do this she will have found a way for both mother and daughter to grow closer together as grown-up friends, in a new relationship that accepts that both are now adult. Only then can the new grandmother be of real help and contribute to her daughter's, son-in-law's and grandchild's happiness.

WHAT IS LIFE FOR?
THE PROBLEM OF THE EX-REVOLUTIONARY

The girl who was active in protest may face special problems when trying to adjust to the idea of having a baby and 'settling down'. It may look to her – and perhaps to her man – as if she is retreating from the world's challenges, and has some-how 'sold out'. She can begin to hate and despise herself and what she thinks she is becoming, in much the same way that the girl previously committed to an exacting job can now feel her life empty and pointless.

She may be aware that she chose pregnancy because at that time she really was seeking a way out, and the temporary mood of depression in which she attempted this escape has now trapped her with a baby. The depression can then become fixed round her like an enveloping jelly from which she cannot break free, and the girl who was before so energetic finds her-self inert, lethargic and withdrawn – passing through a vegeta-tive state of existence which cannot be explained solely in terms of the changed hormone activity of pregnancy. I say 'like a jelly' because it really feels as if there is no barrier to batter against – only an octopus-like stranglehold on action and will.

The girl in this situation particularly needs to be with other women going through the same experience. She has often relied on being a member of a group united for the same purpose, and her sudden isolation leaves her stranded without satisfying human contact. Classes in preparation for childbirth and parenthood can help a great deal because she meets with other expectant mothers.

The couple also need support – because such emotional stresses must be a strain on the relationship, whether it is one of unmarried lovers or of marriage. They need someone to whom they can talk, and the prospective father may need special help to see his role in it all, and how he can express his love for her in this difficult situation.

Couples wanting special help for any of the emotional prob-lems of pregnancy might contact the National Childbirth

Trust,[1] which is often able to put them in touch with an experienced counsellor who has understanding of such problems and, indeed, may have been through them herself.

'FALSE' LABOUR, AND PAINFUL BRAXTON-HICKS CONTRACTIONS

Braxton-Hicks contractions are the 'practice' contractions of the uterus with which it 'rehearses' its role in labour. They take place throughout pregnancy. Not all women are aware of them. There seems to exist no physical reason why they should suddenly become not only much more noticeable but actually distressing. However, a fair proportion of expectant mothers report painful Braxton-Hicks contractions which occur during the last few weeks of pregnancy; others may be so severe and of so rhythmical and recurrent a nature that they feel sure labour is starting. Occasionally, of course, the cervix is already partially dilated before the woman is aware she is in labour, and this may account for these contractions with some women, but the explanation for the majority must be sought in the psychological state of the pregnant woman who is approaching her expected date of confinement – her excitement and anticipation of the event, her longing to 'get on with it', her boredom and irritation with the long-continuing state of pregnancy, the knowledge that friends pregnant at the same time are already delivered, and in some cases the feeling that with every day the baby is growing more and more enormous and therefore more likely to involve her in a difficult labour the longer it is delayed. It is for this reason unwise for the midwife or obstetrician to tell the woman that she 'may have it any day now', that she is 'ready now', and particularly that she is having 'a big baby', since such information can only add to any latent anxiety on this score – and at the back of the minds of many women is a longing for a small baby – even perhaps a little premature, so that labour may be easier.[2]

1. 9 Queensborough Terrace, London W2.
2. A small baby does not necessarily mean a swift, easy labour, however, nor a large baby a painful and protracted one. A woman's preparation and emotional attitude are much more relevant factors.

A woman in the last month of her pregnancy needs gaiety, evidence of affection, tender understanding of her worries from her husband, and the spice of varied social contacts and leisure activities.

BIRTH AS FULFILMENT

Despite the problems of adjustment of both wife and husband, a woman can be happier when she is pregnant than at any other time in her life. It would give a very one-sided picture of pregnancy if one were to concentrate exclusively upon its problems of adjustment and the inner conflicts with which it may be connected. She is often radiant with the new life within her, for which she has secretly longed, even, perhaps, when they were taking precautions against conception. Indeed, I think that contraceptives, used at the beginning of a marriage particularly, can occasionally have an inhibiting effect upon the expression of a woman's desire, not only because they involve conscious planning and forethought, but because some of the wonder of intercourse is taken away if the woman knows that it cannot result in a child. (A similar inhibiting effect is produced, of course, when a couple fail to use an efficient contraceptive technique and are afraid of bearing a child.)

To a man, having children is not an inherent part of sex. The baby does not grow in his body for nine long months, and the cleavage between the act of intercourse and the event of birth is complete for all but the most sensitive men who can imaginatively project themselves into their wives' feelings during pregnancy and childbirth. For a woman, longing for a child can be as disturbing and impelling as sexual desire alone can be for a man. Some women cannot reach orgasm after they have learned that it is impossible for them to have a child.

Few men recall with delight, or even remember, the nights upon which their children were conceived. But women like to be able to think of that particular act of love as a special occasion memorable for the intensity of its passion and the depth of its tenderness. Sometimes if they are not sure when the child was conceived they recreate the occasion in fantasy. From that precious moment the searching sperm entered deep into the woman and sought out the ovum within the darkness and warmth of her body. The gap between conception and birth has for her not only the physical bridge of the growing child moving in her heavy body but is spanned emotionally by this creative fantasy.

Whatever minor discomforts may be involved in pregnancy, this time of preparation is for many women a very happy one, a period in which a woman feels she is being used to the full, bears hope in her body despite all the cruelty and disaster of the world and is sharing in the miracle of new life. During the first four months the baby is not a reality and the woman can hardly believe that she is pregnant, but once she feels the quickening she begins to know and to recognize her child and to form a relationship with him, even though he may prove rather different when born from what she expected. In the later months of pregnancy she conducts, as it were, a two-way conversation, with the world outside, and with the baby within her. She responds to communication coming from two different directions. The fact that she establishes this relationship with her baby *in utero* does not mean that she is self-centred. The baby is so obviously other than herself, and she and her husband may even address him jokingly by name. As her body ripens and term approaches, the reality of the experience which confronts her, its inescapability and its inevitability, sometimes threaten her composure and she needs moral support from those who can describe labour as something wonderful in itself, and not just something to be lived through for the sake of having the baby. But the bravest women approach it with something like timidity, even if it is a timidity born of awe rather than fear, for they are on the threshold of the unknown.

CHAPTER 4

Learning Harmony in Labour: Relaxation

The same stream of life that runs through my veins night and day
runs through the world and dances in rhythmic measure. It is the
same life that shoots in joy through the dust of the earth in number-
less waves of grass and breaks into tumultuous waves of leaves and
flowers. It is the same life that is rocked in the ocean-cradle of birth
and of death, in ebb and in flow. I feel my limbs are made glorious
by the touch of this world of life. And my pride is from the life-
throb of ages dancing in my blood this moment.

RABINDRANATH TAGORE, *Gitanjali,* lxix

THE aim of the exercises described in the next three chapters
is to help a woman understand herself and her body better.
None of the techniques are intended, for example, to be
used to distract a woman from her labour. It is not a training
aimed at occupying her mind with irrelevant physical activities simply to divert attention from sensations coming from
the cervix. Every technique which she learns is essentially an
adaptive one, and is designed to help her relate herself better
to her body. She neither concentrates on a tune, for example,
in order not to 'notice' the intensity of the contraction, nor
thinks of subjects far removed from the reality which she is
experiencing, whether this be a sunny seashore or a diagram
intended to represent a labour contraction (but which is, in
fact, very far removed from anything a contraction *feels* like).
There is nothing to escape from, nothing to deny, nothing she
cannot face.

Nor is the aim simply a mechanical drill in which a woman
says to herself, 'One, two, three, contract. One, two, three,
relax.' Exercising at this level is probably not much help for
labour. It is much more a question of what she thinks and
feels about her body in relation to the actual tensions and the
subsequent release from tension that she is increasingly able
to observe, a matter of the way she 'sees' her body. A French
psychologist has said that 'relaxation is not simply learning

at the level of muscular tone, but involves a maturing of the body image. In other words we simply cannot think of relaxation as a more or less specialized form of gymnastics, but must see it as an emotional experience involving a human being as an existential whole (embracing past, present and future).'[1]

Stanislavski, the great actor and producer, understood this. And in the acting system which he created he was concerned with developing outward action from what he called 'inner truth', from the very core of the person, the identity of each role that an actor must seek to understand and to interpret. For instance he said on one occasion:

In order to differentiate silk and velvet one needs another tempo and rhythm than in differentiating the bristles of a clothes brush. To smell ammonia one needs another tempo and rhythm than in smelling lilies of the valley. If one smells ammonia as one smells lilies of the valley, with rapid breathings-in of various duration and rhythm, one runs the risk of burning the whole mucous membrane of the nose. In a series of variegated exercises I tried to develop in my pupils not the outward rhythm of movement and action, but the inner rhythm of that unseen energy which calls out movement and action. In this manner I was able to develop in my pupils the sensation of movement and gesture, walking, and the entire inner pulse of life.[2]

In this chapter the reader will find a new approach to relaxation which, although it is based on Jacobson's teaching, goes beyond this and uses both techniques inspired by the Method school of acting and experiments in 'body-language' and touch. This can be useful in helping her to come to terms with her body and to understand it better as she is swept through the enormous physical and emotional changes of pregnancy, labour and motherhood. This training is not so far removed from the facts of labour as it may seem at first sight. In becoming more aware of her relationship with her body in its manifest functions, a woman acquires a skill which permits her to remain in control of her labour, but, more than this – allows her to go *with* it, to surrender herself

1. B. This, *Revue de médecine psychosomatique,* vol. 3, No. 2, 1961 (my translation).
2. Constantin Stanislavski, *My Life in Art,* Bles, 1924.

to it, to answer the stimuli coming from her cervix with adaptive behaviour of her whole body and her breathing rhythms. The 'muscle-bound' woman determined to do well, to put all she has learned into practice, to forget no part of her drill, is perhaps the one least likely to have a simple, smoothly functioning labour.

The ability to relax is not, as is sometimes thought, only an inherent characteristic, born in some people but of which others are deprived. It can be acquired with practice and concentration, and some of those who think they are least able to relax and say that they never will be, relax better than those who face life generally with less apparent tension and who seem to have sleepier sorts of natures. Time and time again I have seen emotionally taut, intelligent, self-critical and persevering women teach their bodies how to relax, controlling them with their minds, and acquiring a skill which is useful to them not only in labour but whenever they find themselves tense in their daily lives.

So often in routine tasks about the home and office, muscles are contracted unnecessarily, and the efficient performance of an action is thereby reduced and energy wasted. If a woman observes herself carefully when she is beating eggs, polishing shoes, writing a letter or typing, she will probably discover that she is tensing her shoulders, compressing her abdomen, gritting her teeth, holding her breath, or doing any of a number of things which give clear indication that she is not allowing her energy to flow naturally and easily into the task she is performing, and is making difficulties for herself in the smooth performance of that action. It takes a little self-observation to check oneself in these unnecessary muscular contractions, and the first stage in learning relaxation is the cultivation of the ability to be conscious of them.

Even so, some women protest that they cannot relax 'properly' – that they cannot allow their minds to drift and to become a blank, and their bodies to sink into a sort of semi-slumber. Women who feel this way need not think they are rare cases. Most of us lead lives that are too busy and have minds that are too active for this sort of trance-like relaxation.

If a woman feels wound up like a watch-spring when she tries to relax she should use the activity of her mind to enable her to focus and concentrate upon the control of certain specific muscles and groups of muscles. She can think not in terms of passively submitting to a state of relaxation but of actively *stripping off tension*.

Exercise 1

Lie down comfortably with all joints well flexed and with plenty of cushions wherever you want them, in an airy but warm room (a cold atmosphere makes muscles contract), and close your eyes. Feel them as heavy lidded. Feel the whole eye as heavy. Listen to the sound of your own breathing, and with each breath out concentrate upon stripping off muscular tension wherever you are aware of it. Feel the shoulder-blades as if they were opening outwards, like a dress that is slipping off a hanger at both ends. Contract the abdominal muscles and then feel the easy release as you relax them. Feel the chest as tight all round, and then consciously release those muscles so that it expands loosely with each breath out. Breathe in and out for a little while like this until you are quite sure that respiration is effortless and full.

Now make the breath out a little longer – as long as you can comfortably make it. Breathe in through your nose and out through your mouth, emphasizing the breath out and *relaxing a little more with each breath out*; let the breath in look after itself. Feel as if you are breathing right down your back. If you have good back support, all the way up from the bottom of your spine to the top of your head, which includes support in the small of the back and behind the neck, you will feel a slight, almost imperceptible movement along the length of the spine as you breathe. After all, it is constructed more like a string of sausages than a lamp-post; breathe steadily and rhythmically and note the faint movement of the vertebrae as you continue breathing in and out. *Use* your breathing to relax further.

Are there any points at which you are still tense? You will help yourself if you can think of them as warm, as if you have just had a hot water bottle there. If this is insufficient a hot water bottle (not too hot) actually resting behind your shoulders or between your legs or wherever it is that you are still tense will help. Once you have got the idea of feeling the muscles warm you will be able to *imagine* them warm and so release them consciously. Feel your whole scalp warm as if you have just come out from under a hair dryer, warm and tingling.

Feel each limb heavy, every bone heavy, the pull of gravity drawing your body down to the earth. Allow your knees to flop apart, your whole body feel as if it is melting.

Now all this is much easier if you have someone, your husband, or a friend with whom you do not feel self-conscious, to read it out aloud to you once you have had an initial try yourself in privacy, and to test your relaxation as you proceed. It is reassuring to know that you really are achieving something, and only too easy to *think* that one is relaxed when, in fact, one is very far from it. Your husband can pick up a hand and let it drop, noting if there is any resistance. He should be able smoothly and slowly to move your hand in circles from the wrist, your arm at the elbow, and, holding your hand, your arm at the shoulder, without feeling that any of the works need oiling. If he is tempted to criticize your performance or to get impatient, see if he can relax. It is not so easy. His criticism should always be positive and constructive. After the hand and arm, he tests your legs. First with a hand under the ankle he lifts the leg from the knee and lets it drop. Then, once there is no resistance, he bends one leg so that the knee is raised towards the abdomen, and then moved in a circle. Make sure that the muscle running along the inside of the upper leg, the adductor, is well released, or this can be uncomfortable.

If you are lying with your head fairly low and really well relaxed he can hold your toes and shake them firmly and gently, and you will shake all the way up to your head, which wobbles on top like one of those Japanese wooden dolls. (Of course all this is slightly ridiculous and I hope that you will find yourselves laughing about it. It should not be taken dead seriously. Laughter helps you to relax.)

He puts a hand on either side of the pelvis, that is, low on your hips, and gently and firmly rocks you from side to side. He holds your head in his hands and does the same, lifting the chin up and down and rocking the head also towards the chest and up again. You feel your head warm and heavy, like a great glass ball.

When you get up after lying relaxed always have a good stretch and see if you can make yourself yawn. Get up slowly, gradually unfolding yourself, like Cleopatra rising from her barge, if you can conjure up this image in pregnancy! If you jump straight up you may feel giddy.

Exercise 2

We are aiming to relax more completely by degrees. So in order to proceed to phase 2 in the study of neuro-muscular release, you will have to go back to the beginning, and do Exercise 1 again, in careful detail.

When you are well relaxed begin to think especially about the muscles of your face. Our moods and thoughts are quickly reflected in our faces. Every muscle can respond to the emotions of joy, grief, tenderness, love or hate.

Concentrate first on the cheeks. Feel them warm and rosy. As you breathe in, allow your nostrils to dilate slightly, and let the breathing movement spread across your cheeks. Let your lips part slightly, smooth and soft, as if you have just put on a new and expensive lipstick! The tip of the tongue rests against the inside of the front lower teeth. The tongue is broad and soft.

The jaw is relaxed; let it go at the point where it joins the skull just in front of the ears. Think of the eyelids heavy; imagine you are wearing a heavy double row of fur eyelashes. Feel the space between the eyes getting wider and wider. Your brow is smooth and broad. Your face is now relaxed.

Exercise 3

Do exercises 1 and 2 and then proceed to exercises which will help you to develop an awareness of tensions around and behind the eyes themselves.

Let your eyes close.

Imagine that there is a ship sailing away from you and that you are watching it move towards the distant horizon. Follow its course carefully; keep your eyes on it; watch it sail on and on, and then dip over the horizon. Relax your eyes entirely.

Imagine that you have a newspaper in front of you with a photograph of the Queen. Focus your eyes upon it. Then relax.

Now spread out this imaginary newspaper and start to read it, and you will feel the pull of the eye muscles from left to right and back to the beginning of the line. Relax.

See a large six-storey building in front of you and watch a fireman hoist a ladder and climb slowly to the top storey. You will feel a different sort of muscular pull as your eyes move in a different direction. Now watch him slowly coming down again. He is at the bottom. Rest your eyes.

You are watching a tennis match. Without moving your head,

keep your eye on the ball. Note the muscle tension. Now rest your eyes, and you will experience a release from tension which is very pleasant. Now your eyes are relaxed.

See mentally a vivid scarlet, green and white detergent advertisement just in front of you. You may almost feel your eyes recoil from it, since it gives a visual shock. Now look into the far distance, at blue-hazed mountains, very still in the morning air. You will feel relief as the strain on the eyes disappears.

You can do these same exercises with your eyes open, learning how to release unnecessary tension even while keeping your eyes open. All this is important in labour. Although you may find it helps to concentrate on relevant visual imagery then – the stretching cervix, or the baby as it moves towards the outside world – your eyes should be relaxed.

Exercise 4

Do Exercises 1 and 2 first. Then proceed to abdominal contraction and relaxation. Pull in the abdominal wall strongly towards the spine. Hold it for fifteen seconds or so, and then relax. Let yourself spread. Relax all round, not only the very front of the abdomen, but the sides too – all round the barrel as it were.

Now imagine that you are pulling on a girdle – an old-fashioned heavy-boned thick rubber type – that is three sizes too small. Act the movements, and really feel the effort to get it up over your thighs, buttocks, the bulge in front and, at last, on up to the waist. Now you have to do up six hooks and eyes at the side. Pull hard. Notice what is happening to your breathing. On top of the hooks there is a zip, and you know how painful it is when bare flesh catches in a zip, so do this very carefully. This is contraction of the abdominal muscles. And now: relax! Now *that* is abdominal relaxation!

Once you are relaxed, notice the sensation. This is how the abdominal muscles will be throughout labour, as you do not need to use them then.

Exercise 5

Do Exercises 1, 2 and 4. Now relax for a minute or so, enjoying the sheer luxury of it. Then proceed to contraction and relaxation of the muscles around the chest and shoulders. In labour all these will be released, and it is very difficult to do the different levels and rates of breathing well unless they are well relaxed. Any tension makes for greater difficulty with breathing, especially with the shallower quick breathing. Imagine that you are putting on a bra three sizes too small. You have just had a bath and your skin is still rather damp. Lift yourself into it and then pull hard; go on pulling; you are not nearly there yet. Try harder. Notice what is happening to your breathing and to the muscles of your face. Rest completely and feel the luxury of relaxation after effort.

Exercise 6

Do Exercises 1, 2, 4 and 5. Then remove the support under your knees. Lie with knees bent and soles of the feet flat on the bed or floor near your buttocks. Place a hand on each leg just up inside the knees. Tightening the muscles along the insides of the legs, pull your knees towards each other against the resistance of your hands. Pull hard till the knees are pointing up stiffly towards the ceiling. Then let them flop out again and relax. Tighten the muscles just at the top of the left leg, pulling the knee in and up again, and relax. Now just the right leg, and relax.

Press the legs out away from each other progressively, resisting their movement with hands placed outside the upper thighs. Feel the stretch and pull along the adductors. Relax them completely.

Exercise 7

Do Exercises 1, 2, 4, 5 and 6.

Now check to see if you are able to contract some muscles whilst keeping the rest of your body relaxed. This is 'differential' relaxation. It is the basis of all efficient harmonious activity in which energy is not wasted and only the minimum of tension required for the task is called upon.

Lying on your back on the floor with pillows where you require them, and with your bent knees resting on pillows, tense the calf muscle of one leg, without tensing anywhere else in your body. Do not raise the leg, or you will be pulling on abdominal muscles. Practise this until you are quite sure that there is no unnecessary tension anywhere. Then relax completely. Now do it with the other leg, relax, and then with both legs. Relax.

Now raise one arm a little from the floor, like a wooden doll, with the fist clenched, but allow the legs to remain relaxed, and check that you are not tensing any other muscles or holding your breath. Keep the position for a few seconds and then release the arm and let it sink back on to the floor or bed. Do it with the other arm, relax. Then try it with both arms at once, and relax.

This time contract the calf muscle of one leg and the arm on the same side, keeping the other leg and the other arm perfectly relaxed. Be sure that your face is not tensing with concentration. Hold the tension for a little, and then relax, and do it with the other arm and leg. And relax.

Now try it with the arm and a leg on opposite sides. Make sure that the tension is not spreading across your body, and that you are not contracting abdominal muscles. Contract only the arm and the leg. Now relax, and do it with the other arm and leg. Relax.

In all these phases of differential relaxation it is a great help if someone will check the limbs that should be relaxed. If you get cramp in your legs, however, adapt this exercise so that you do not contract muscles in your legs.

DEVISING YOUR OWN EXERCISES

Once you have reached this stage of learning relaxation, and not only relaxation, but a much more intricate and subtle awareness of your body, you are ready to start using your imagination and ability to remember patterns of contractions in different everyday situations involving stress, to evolve exercises of your own based on the tensions which you personally are inclined to have. That is, you start with simple actions, as when you pull open a heavy drawer which has stuck, push a door which has caught on the carpet, or open the kitchen door with one hand whilst balancing a tray in the other. Having observed and isolated them, the next task is to re-create these particular contractions, as you lie down practising your relaxation. This particular set of exercises can even be done in the bath. Always relax *between* exercises of this kind or you find that you carry over residual tension from the last one.

Here are a few suggestions, to which you will be able to add many:

You have a mouth full of neat lemon juice. Relax.

You are breathing in the fumes from an open bottle of ammonia. Relax. It is gone!

You are walking on the beach, barefoot, with sharp jagged pebbles under your feet. Pick your way carefully up the beach. Then relax.

You are carrying a large, heavy, precious crystal bowl. It is wet and belongs to someone else. Wearing high heels, you carry it across a slippery kitchen floor. Feel the tension in your hands as they curve round the bowl, in the arms and shoulders, and in the eyes, since you must watch it. Put it down carefully, and relax.

You are walking along a thin, white line, balancing one foot carefully in front of the other. You feel tension in the arches of the feet, the toes, the thighs, the buttocks, the lower back, and also in the arms, hands and shoulders, and you strive to keep your balance. Relax completely.

You are getting into an icy cold Scottish loch, toes first. Let the cold water steal up your legs, over the abdomen; gradually sink right under the water, feeling it rise up your back. Now get out and throw yourself on a warm beach in the sun. Feel the sand hot under your body, the sun pouring into your skin, warm air all over the surface of the skin. Visualize yourself falling into a deep, restful sleep lying there. Stand outside yourself, as it were, and see your body lying there in the hot sunlight, breathing peacefully, perfectly relaxed.

If you are a car driver, imagine a situation in which you are about to overtake, and then notice another car overtaking and coming towards you. Notice the specific tensions that result in the eyes, arms, shoulders, and the leg with which you step on the brake. Now feel this tension 'uncoil', and relax completely.

Imagine that you are stooping down to get a heavy casserole out of a very hot oven. You have filled it too full, and the gravy is slopping over. Feel the contraction of muscles as you squat down; turn the handle of the oven door; start back as the heat comes into your face, and then carefully, holding an oven cloth, lean forward and take this large casserole out. You will be aware of a whole series of tensions in these movements, involving muscles in the back, the feet and legs, the hands, neck, face and arms. Now let all this tension go.

To observe contractions associated with muscles involved in speech, lying perfectly relaxed say your husband's name out loud. Notice the contraction of jaw muscles, and others in the face, particularly around the mouth. Maybe if you are feeling cross with him at the moment, other muscles are involved too – reflecting the tension you feel about him. Relax completely. Now say his name again, in a whisper. Notice the contraction of the same muscles, but less strongly. Relax. Now simply *think* of saying his name. If you are very observant you may notice slight contraction of the very same muscles. So even imagined physical activity of a minimal nature is reflected in muscular contraction. (Perhaps this is one of the reasons why it is so tiring to lie in bed *thinking* about getting up in the morning!)

You can devise a number of imaginary activities for yourself in this way, and observe the specific tensions that each involves. As you stop each one, you will know what it feels like to strip the tension from these particular muscles.

See if you can benefit from this awareness to use only the necessary muscle contractions in your everyday life, so avoiding the stresses which come from wasted muscle energy.

Situations involving emotional conflict

From there you move on to less common situations of stress, and to those involving emotional conflict. Here you begin to draw on your personal experience of life – tensions which, perhaps, nobody else is aware of. Try to be honest with yourself and to note and analyse them carefully. None of us goes through life cool, calm and collected all of the time. In a book I can only throw out a few hints and suggestions, basing these on tensions many women experience.

Do not attempt to recreate an emotion in yourself without recreating the *specific circumstances* which lead up to the expression of this emotion, or what you do will be forced and artificial. 'Don't think about the feeling itself, but set your mind to work on what makes it grow, what the conditions were that brought about the experience. . . . *Never begin with results. They will appear in time as the logical outcome of what has gone before.*'[1]

1. Constantin Stanislavski, *An Actor Prepares,* Bles, 1937.

You are whisking cream in a hurry, with your mother-in-law just about to come into the kitchen.

You are waiting at the booking-office for your ticket and the train is just about to leave.

Walking down a lonely country lane at night (it is pitch dark) you think you hear someone walking behind you. He seems to be creeping in the shadow of the hedge. Did you hear a noise? Notice your reactions. How was your breathing affected?

You are lying in bed at night desperately wanting to cry and not wanting your husband to notice how unhappy you are. (In point of fact, maybe this is an unfamiliar one for you. But try it all the same. Most women have to kick their husbands awake before they notice that anything is wrong!) Notice the tightness of your face – like a mask – the tensed abdominal muscles, the dry feeling in the throat, and the effect on your breathing. What other muscles are contracted?

Now concentrate on situations and things that you really worry about or fear. Sometimes these fears are irrational, occasionally reasonable. Make a list (you can burn it afterwards) of those subjects which involve great stress, which worry you deeply, or of which you are afraid. Include anything to do with your baby, pregnancy, the hospital, your marriage, or the way your body works. Perhaps the list is small – do not artificially manufacture fears – but it will still provide material for practice.

Select one subject and give your imagination free rein so that it is vivid and real for you to work on. You are going to re-live the tensions associated with it, whether it is a mouse running along the floor, someone staying in the house who causes unhappiness, your toddler almost knocked down by a car, the empty house at night with the door creaking, or things like the pain of a menstrual period or a miscarriage, being constipated, an asthma attack or migraine, painful love-making, or even having a tooth stopped at the dentist's (but in this case start off analysing your tensions in the waiting-room).

Imagine yourself looking out over the edge of a high building, or shut in the cupboard under the stairs; think of a situation in which you have become so worked up that you felt like bursting with rage – those few seconds before you struck out or screamed or fled; think perhaps of a particularly unpleasant dream that has been haunting you – the knife edge, the locked cupboard or narrow passage, squirming snakes or crawling insects, being tied down on an operating table, on the edge of a precipice, drowning, or bearing a monster child. (Most women seem to have intensified, uncomfortable dreams in pregnancy.) Really act it, and once you are living the part, stand outside yourself and observe yourself in it. What muscles are contracted? How are you breathing? Where is the tension concentrated?

Now consciously, deliberately, send a message from your brain to the muscles involved – rather like a telephone message – switching the contractions off. Relax completely.

Now summon up the picture again, repeat the exercise. Switch off the contractions instantaneously when you wish to relax.

Summon up the picture again, and this time *meet* it with relaxation instead of tension. This may be difficult at first. You will acquire skill as you practise.

Gradually you will develop a new neuro-muscular awareness – quite different from intellectual knowledge about your body. It will be useful to you not only in labour, but in every situation in which you react with tension – and is a firm basis on which to build more specific relaxation for labour. Controlled relaxation derived from an understanding of yourself and your personal reactions is the starting point. When you have achieved this you are already half way along the road.

TOUCH RELAXATION

Another approach to relaxation can be made through touch, and best of all the touch of a woman by the man she loves, and the following exercises are designed to increase awareness of body tensions and release, and also to be a pleasure in themselves. They can be done in bed, and preferably with no or few clothes on. This method can be useful for those women who find the imaginative exercises we have just been doing difficult because they seem unable to visualize the situations easily. But ideally the student should try different approaches to relaxation and aim at being expert with them all.

The aim of touch relaxation is to by-pass words and to try to use other forms of stimulus. To do this we aim at building up a non-verbal communication based on touch.

Not everyone relaxes in response to the same sort of stimulus and methods of teaching relaxation ought to be as varied as the women to whom we try to teach it. In my own teaching of relaxation I have found it useful to experiment with a wide range of verbal imagery, and to attempt all the time to adapt my teaching to what appear to me to be the needs of each particular woman. Even the best sort of image may fail dismally for a woman with whom, because of her personal experience and memories, the words conjure up a situation which is either unknown, or preposterous, or un-comfortable: I remember suggesting that complete release of muscles of the scalp felt as if one's head was warm – as if one had just come out from under the hair dryer, and a student flinched at the thought, and protested, 'But I can't *bear* that! I *hate* that feeling!' The teacher therefore needs to be aware of the response in each particular instance, and at the same time be developing, with the help of her students, new images and a store of relevant similes.

So we need not depend upon verbal stimuli alone. Our culture is, or has been up till now, a highly verbal one, and we tend to teach through and with words when sometimes there are other means of communication open to us, and means of communication which we need not leave to chance or spon-taneous impulse – such as when we smile or lean forward, or reach out a hand.[1] Non-verbal methods of communication, which are taking place all the time alongside the purely verbal methods, and which may intrude on and actually alter the message of verbal communication, can themselves be ex-

1. See, for example, Michael Argyle: *The Psychology of Interpersonal Be-baviour* (Penguin) and the works of R. D. Laing.

amined, analysed and structured so that we can use them deliberately, with forethought and skill.

I have been experimenting recently with using non-verbal means of communication as a systematized method of instruction in neuro-muscular release, and I have found this simplest to base on the quite spontaneous way in which husband and wife touch each other, because they like to, and because it gives them pleasure, comfort, reassurance, erotic delight and companionship. I have an abhorrence of the sort of antenatal exercise which entails putting on leotards and leaping around doing a parade-ground drill for 'B day', and although I realize that some women find it very cheering I cannot see how, apart from pepping up the circulation, it can have any possible effect on a woman's effective adaptive responses during labour.

But labour, anyway, is not the be-all and end-all of life, and to practise only with the few hours of labour in mind is to limit our teaching of relaxation unnecessarily. After the birth, what then? The woman is holding a baby in her arms. And how does she hold it? When she is feeding the baby, and changing it and bathing it, and when she holds her toddler, or greets her mother-in-law, or copes in the kitchen or does her housework, writes her thesis, or deals with illness in the family, when she is driving a car, or shopping, or offering help to someone in distress, or dealing with all the maddening, chaotic, nerve-wracking, ear-splitting crises in a family ... how is she then? Of course the answer is that we scream and weep and shake our children till their teeth chatter, and we get headaches and all sorts of psychosomatic illnesses, and we say things we wish to heaven we hadn't said, and then we feel guilty because we have done all these things; we make valiant efforts to improve, prayer or meditation over the washing-up perhaps, uplifting passages from Spock in the dressing-table drawer, earnest discussion with other equally guilty mums. This is how I am anyway, and it is because I know my own besetting sins that I feel relaxation should be tackled at the level of ordinary, everyday living and be something we can incorporate into life, rather than an 'exercise'.

The basic grammar of this non-verbal language of touch is simple – release *towards* the touching hand. This is what you do spontaneously when someone you love touches you. At the same time it is important that the husband learns that he should touch with a relaxed hand, slowly, moulding his hand to the shape of the limb or any other part of the body on which the couple is working. Thus it is a mutual exercise in release, and there is never a question of the wife becoming a criticized pupil – subordinate to the husband; instead they are participating together in what is really not so much an exercise as a 'sensitivity response'.

The woman contracts a set of muscles, and when she is ready (not before) he rests his hand on the contracted muscles. At the second he does so, she releases towards his hand. There are various ways in which this can be done, and it is a good idea to concentrate on parts of the body which the woman finds it rather more difficult to relax. She lies on her back, propped up and well supported with pillows in a warm bed, with support all up her spine, including the small of her back and back of her neck, and under her knees. She breathes out and relaxes completely. One system of exploring ease of release over different parts of the body is as follows:

1. She frowns. He rests his hand on her brow. She relaxes.
2. She grits her teeth and clenches her jaw. He rests his hands on either side of her jaw. She relaxes.
3. She contracts muscles of the scalp and raises her eyebrows. He rests his hands on either side of the scalp. She relaxes.
4. She presses her shoulder-blades back as if they were angel's wings and she could make them touch each other. He rests his hands at the front of each shoulder. She relaxes.
5. She pulls in her abdominal wall towards her spine. He rests his hands on the curve of her abdomen. She relaxes.
6. She presses her upper legs together 'as if you could hold a sheet of paper between them'. He touches the outside of each leg. She relaxes and her legs flop apart.
7. She presses her legs out, still flexed, but forcing her

thighs apart. He rests his hands on the inside thighs, and she relaxes.

8. She contracts the muscles of her right arm like a wooden doll. He first rests his hand on her clenched fist, and her hand relaxes from the wrist. Then slowly he runs both hands up the arm on either side to the elbow and she relaxes her forearm as he does so. He then moves up to her shoulder and presses firmly on it, and by this time her whole arm is relaxed.

9. Repeat with the other arm.

10. She contracts the muscles of one leg by pointing the toes up towards the ceiling and straightening the leg (this should not be done if it causes cramp). He touches her bare foot firmly round the instep (if he does not do it firmly he will tickle her). She relaxes the foot from the ankle. Then, slowly and deliberately, he moves his hands up the leg to the knee, on either side, until she is relaxed from the knee down. Then he moves up to the top of the leg, and by this time her whole leg is released.

11. Repeat with the other leg.

The woman then turns on her side or in the front lateral, whichever is the most comfortable, and in this position:

12. She raises her chin in the air and contracts muscles at the back of the neck. He rests a hand in the nape of her neck and she releases.

13. She hollows the small of her back. He rests both hands against either side of the sacro-lumbar spine and she releases.

14. She presses her buttocks together 'as if she had a £5 note between them and someone was trying to take it away'. He rests a hand on each buttock, and she relaxes.

Each of these positions of tension is related to specific common stress situations in which this tends to be the reaction, both in everyday life, and in the different phases of labour.

We often contract muscles of the scalp and back of the neck – as in Exercise 3, for instance – when we have a headache, and sometimes contraction of these muscles in situations of stress appears to precede the onset of a tension headache, and looks as if it might be the cause of the pain. In Exercise 4, contraction of muscles of the shoulders and the top of the back are involved, in just the way that they may be when there is a build-up of tension in the late first stage of labour. Contraction of these muscles is very likely to result in over-breathing and consequent hyper-ventilation of the maternal bloodstream, which we shall see more about when we discuss breathing in labour. The initial effect is to make breathing more difficult; it becomes forced and hectic, and light, easy breathing gives way to heavy panting. The cause is not so much that the breathing is wrong, but that the woman has become tense and is no longer able to breathe gently.

Exercises 6 and 7 give an idea of both the sort of tension that can build up in transition, the difficulty in relaxing which the mother may encounter when she finds her legs get extremely cold and start to shake, as they often do just at the onset of the second stage before she begins pushing, and the way in which she can consciously and carefully relax them.

In Exercise 8 one can get an idea of the sort of help that the husband can give simply by touch in labour. He can use his hand to help his wife relax, and this is more likely to assist her than to encourage her to cling on to his hand. For this reason it is a good idea actually during contractions in labour to hold her by the wrist rather than to grip her hand, and then to use a stroking touch over the muscles of the arm up to the shoulder to help to remind her of the need for complete release. Sometimes a woman does not like being touched at all and wants to be left alone because she finds contact irritating, and obviously each couple must work out what is best for them and what they personally want to do at that time.

Exercise 12 depicts the woman who in the second stage of labour bears down using her throat muscles and strains excessively in a frantic effort to push the baby out. This can be corrected in the same way as in the second part of the exercise, by firm touch at the back of the neck which reminds her to release her neck muscles and to let her chin drop forward on to her chest.

It is during the expulsive stage that many women feel

despair, and unable to make headway, and start to contract muscles in the back, lifting the small of the back away from the delivery table or bed. This again can be corrected with firm pressure of the husband's hand against this part of her back.

In Exercise 14 we get a picture of a woman who is resisting the odd sensations of pressure. This can make her feel as if the baby is coming out of the 'wrong hole' and that she is going to pop. The foetal head descends through the birth canal, feels as if it fills the rectum and anus, and later spreads open the vagina. Both the adductors inside the upper legs, and glutei, or buttock muscles, may contract if the mother is fighting these sensations.

So touch relaxation techniques can also find a place actually in labour, and are a valuable means of the husband offering practical labour support, which neither involves nagging nor puts the woman into the situation where she feels: 'Who's having this baby – you or me?'

The husband who is alert and sensitive to see the build-up of tension, however slight, can rest his hand on muscles involved, both between contractions, and, if the wife wishes it, at the onset of contractions. Here there must be ability to communicate easily, since touch can also be an intrusion, and should only be used in labour when the woman finds it really helpful. Massage is a logical extension of touch relaxation, and there is more about this on page 108.

It should be emphasized that once a woman has become skilful she can (a) use her own touch, too, to assist release, and (b) accept the touch of doctor and midwife also as a signal for release, although their touch is primarily exploratory and is not aimed at providing the same stimulus. Once a woman, previously tense, can discover the effect of releasing when the obstetrician examines her, and instead of 'drawing in her horns like a snail' can relax completely, the increased comfort she experiences, and her doctor's surprise, provides its own impetus to perfecting relaxation for labour.

RELAXING IN LABOUR

Contraction of a muscle in any part of the body is rather like the contraction of the uterus in labour. In each case there is a shortening and drawing-up of muscle fibre, and a similar use of energy. Of course, the uterus has to contract, or there would be no labour. But you do not need to use contractions in the rest of your body. In fact, unnecessary contractions can only make labour more tiring and uncomfortable, and even make it longer.

If you clench your fist, holding your arm up, for a few minutes, you will notice an ache coming in the muscles concerned as they are involved in unusual contraction. In a similar way the uterus often aches, especially around the cervix, as the longitudinal muscle fibres are contracted and the cervix is gradually opened.

There is however a basic difference between the ache that you bring about in the biceps and the contraction of the uterus. The biceps are controlled voluntarily by your mind. The uterus, like the heart, operates independently of thinking and willing, and goes on working without your needing to do anything about it.[1] In fact, the uterus has contractions throughout a woman's child-bearing life, although she is usually unaware of them. As pregnancy continues the contractions increase in intensity and frequency so that they can even be felt by someone with a hand on your abdomen. During most of labour the actual pressure resulting from contractions is not much greater than that during the last weeks of pregnancy, although you will in fact feel them much more.

During the first stage of labour, when the slow thinning out

1. Here we are on territory still to be more fully explored. In *Clinical Measurements of Uterine Forces in Pregnancy and Labour* by S. R. M. Reynolds, Jerome Harris and Irwin H. Kaiser, Charles C. Thomas, Illinois, 1954, an experiment is described in which pills – any pills, providing they did not contain oxytocic substances – were given to pregnant women who were reported 'quite unaware of the uterine activity', and the patients were told that this would 'quieten them down'. The result was that uterine activity was reduced by as much as fifty per cent. We do not yet know the full effect that the mind can have on the uterus.

and subsequent dilatation of the cervix is taking place, all those muscles which can be controlled by the brain should be relaxed so that the muscles of the uterus which are pulling up the opening can work undisturbed. When a woman is truly relaxed, not only is she unaware of any tension – and careful practice of progressive relaxation in the manner described above will help her to detect and to check tension without difficulty – but she begins to feel as if her body is spreading sideways and flowing out of its boundaries rather like a very ripe Camembert. She cannot arrive at this state by willing herself to achieve it, but it is a by-product of her skill in relaxing the separate sets of muscles in her body, and when she feels like this she will know that she has succeeded.

This relaxation can be practised once or twice a day for ten minutes or so at a time, and always on going to bed at night, when it will help to ensure sound, restful sleep. If the woman nearing full term uses this time to think about being in labour and to visualize the physiological processes which she has learned occur during the first and second stages of labour, and to look forward to the experience whilst in this state of neuro-muscular release, she will also be allowing herself the additional aid derived from controlled auto-suggestion.

After each period of neuro-muscular release she should stretch fully once or twice, like a cat in front of a fire, letting energy flow through all her muscles, yawn widely with a deep breath in and a long sigh out, and then get up slowly. In this way she will not only avoid any giddiness from too sudden a movement but will feel greatly refreshed and re-invigorated.

Relaxation should be practised in various different positions. Although a woman may learn to relax in the front lateral position and lying on her back with the knees drawn up, it is important to be able to relax in any other position in which she may find herself when in labour.

If she has to drive to hospital she should practise relaxation in the car. I know one woman who drove to hospital on the back of a motor-bike, relaxing well whilst using a sufficient degree of muscular tension to sit firmly on the machine and not fall off. One mother who came to my classes was an aero-

plane pilot, and flew up till the date of her delivery; she practised relaxation in the small space afforded in the cockpit, just
in case she should start labour when in the air. Another
woman suffered from severe heartburn at the end of pregnancy; she found it much easier to sit up, and practised relaxing like this, which was useful for her, as her heartburn
persisted throughout the first stage of labour, and she found
it impossible to lie down.

If labour proceeds rapidly the woman may find that she is
busy getting things ready at a point when she must yet concentrate upon contractions and break off her activity to cope
with them. In this case it is helpful to be able to relax the
necessary muscles while standing. Some women find it useful
to lean slightly forward with their legs apart and their elbows
resting on a shelf or table, and feel the lower part of the body
go limp. Others like to lean forward with the finger-tips
resting on a piece of furniture. Some find themselves swaying
slightly forward and backward with a rocking movement of
the pelvis during contractions in this position. Some like to
squat down with the pelvis at its widest. Whatever position a
woman chooses to adopt, there is no hard-and-fast rule about
what she should do. The position in which she is most comfortable is the right one for her.

The relaxation that is needed in labour is of the kind that is
required to perform any sport, to dance, to play the piano, to
drive a car or to ride a bicycle. That is, all unnecessary tension
is eliminated, everything that is not required for the task in
hand. One does not, however, collapse in a heap on the floor
or render oneself unconscious to one's environment, going
into a sort of trance and being out of touch with those who
are there to help. The mother can be fully aware of all that
is going on, mentally alert and in control of the situation, and
quick to respond to assistance and guidance coming from her
attendants. Above all, she should remain able to regulate her
breathing. As each contraction comes, she begins the controlled breathing that will enable her to keep abreast of her
labour, and to enjoy its excitement and the energy which is
released in her body.

MASSAGE

Massage is most effective when it is rehearsed beforehand by husband and wife. The first thing for the husband to remember is that all the massage for labour should be done with a relaxed hand (so it is no good him getting too tense about the labour) and the wife should always remember to relax *towards* the massaging hands, so this sort of help becomes a joint activity and not something she passively submits to. They can use body lotion, hand cream or talc if they wish. If the husband wears a wedding ring he should remove it or the wife will feel he is equipped with knuckledusters.

It may be useful to practise these four types:

1. *Massage of the sacro-lumbar region.* The wife lies on her front or side. A firm hand, curved to the shape of the small of the back, with pressure on the heel of the hand is needed. It is best done so that the flesh moves over the bone, and is least effective when the hand just makes a slippery stroking movement over a wide area. Every now and again he sweeps the hand down over the sides of the pelvis and over the buttocks. The wife presses the small of her back slightly towards his hand.

2. *Massage of the lower spine.* The wife lies on her front or side. This is an up and down movement over the lower bones of the spine, covering the beginning of the cleft between the buttocks and about 6″ up, and down again. Here the pressure comes more from the fingers, but the husband must avoid pressing the tips of his fingers into her flesh, which can be painful. The wife presses her buttocks slightly back towards his hand.

3. *Kneading the buttocks.* Anyone who has ever made bread will know how to do this one! It consists of firm massage over the buttock muscles with a slow, leisurely movement, and is useful when the baby is pressing low against the rectum to ensure complete release of those muscles of the pelvic floor which are around the anus. The woman is encouraged to release towards the touch.

4. *Upper back massage.* Although the baby is going to emerge from the other end, it is often surprising how firm rubbing of the area around the shoulders can help the woman to relax and to keep her breathing rhythmic and unstrained. Here again, she releases towards the massaging hand.

5. *Massage of the adductors.* Facing his wife, the husband massages the muscles of the inner thigh from knee to perineum firmly and rhythmically, every now and again sweeping his hands over the outside of her thighs. She sits or lies on her back, legs flopped apart, knees out, and releases her muscles consciously *towards* her husband, *including the muscles of the pelvic floor.*

In labour, as the contraction starts, her husband begins firm regular massage of the adductors. This is a highly effective way of gaining control even after it has been lost for a few contractions, and can be extremely useful at the end of the first stage and during transition (the bridge between the first and second stages).

6. *Light abdominal massage.* Many women find it comforting to stroke the area above the dilating cervix with one hand during contractions, and this can be done by the husband too, provided he remembers to keep a very light touch.

CHAPTER 5

Learning Harmony in Labour: Breathing

WHY BREATHE IN A SPECIAL WAY?

IT might be thought that one could safely leave breathing to chance and that most women in labour breathe all right anyway. From studies done by R. St J. Buxton in Bristol, however, it has been found that untrained women in labour frequently flush out too much carbon dioxide from their blood-stream[1] with a resulting reduction in the flow of blood to the baby. Nor does training for birth avoid this problem if women in labour are told to pant heavily, to do deep quick abdominal breathing, or are taught how to breathe rapidly and shallowly but nevertheless, when they are actually in labour, start to gasp and 'huff and puff'. So it is important not only to learn how to breathe in an easy, relaxed, rhythmic way, but to *allow for a margin of error* in the stress of labour, and particularly near full dilatation.

The way in which a woman breathes is closely connected with the rhythm to which her body adapts itself during the process of labour. If she succeeds in harmonizing her breathing with the contractions of the uterus, which have a definite rhythm of their own and are like waves in the way that they gather, rise to a crest, and then die away, she will be able to keep control of her labour, and instead of its being a muddle of painful sensations she will find it very exhilarating.

Before women have had a child they often think that childbirth entails a great deal of pushing and straining and that therefore the really important purpose of prenatal exercises is that one should develop very strong abdominal muscles. I have even heard of midwives who believed this. But after they have had a baby they realize that it is more a matter of breath-

1. See 'The Aims of Breathing Exercises in Childbirth' in *Physiotherapy*, Vol. 56, No. 12, December 1970.

ing and coordination than of straining and making terrific muscular efforts to expel the baby.

Many women find that the harmony they create between the contractions and their breathing gives them real delight. Even when the contractions are very fierce – at the end of the first stage of labour when the cervix of the uterus is almost fully dilated – by synchronizing the breathing with the rhythm of the contractions it is possible for labour to be pleasurable, much like swimming in a stormy sea.

If a woman tries to resist the uterine contractions, or merely to endure them, she will have severe pain; instead, she must go *with* them and cooperate with them in getting her baby born. As each one comes, therefore, she should *greet it with her breathing*.

The teaching of Lamaze and Vellay in France taught that learning about breathing and being able to control it can help a woman also by allowing her to get enough oxygen.

But we now know that in fact women very rarely go short of oxygen either in pregnancy or labour, because of an increased tidal volume and more complete expiration, an increased movement of the diaphragm, and increased blood flow which passes more slowly through the lungs, so that there is more time for oxygen to be absorbed. All this means that the labouring woman need not worry about getting enough oxygen, and certainly does not normally need additional oxygen from a mask.

As labour contractions become very forceful at the end of the first stage a woman usually finds it easier to breathe more shallowly and more rapidly than she did earlier in labour, and this often occurs spontaneously, without previous instruction. She has to learn to breathe both shallowly and *rhythmically*, maintaining steady control over inspiration and expiration.

Rhythmic breathing can also help in that it enables the woman to steady herself. It is almost impossible to panic when breathing carefully and concentrating on it. So closely is breathing connected with the emotions that the first signs of fear, frustration, or anger are registered in a changed respiratory rhythm, and just as emotions affect the breathing, so it can work the other way and breathing steadily and carefully can keep one calm and tranquil. Even in normal respiration psychological influence is evident. A woman may have noticed the change in rhythm and the deeper, slower breathing she tends to use when she is concentrating hard on something, the quicker, shallower breathing when she is excited or anticipating something exciting, the irregular arhythmic breathing of surprise. There have been studies made of all these different emotions and their effects on respiration.[1] In so far as adjustment to labour is connected with breathing this has an obvious bearing upon the process of childbirth and one's preparation for it.

Concentrating upon the breathing rhythm also has the effect of centring the woman's attention on something she can actively do to help herself, so that she does not suffer labour passively, but engages positively in constructive adjustment to what is happening in her body. This aspect of the contribution of respiration to childbirth with joy is no less important because it is largely psychological. The mind – not only the uterus – is an important factor in birth.

Breathing correctly probably also helps to alleviate discomfort and pain by preventing unnecessary pressure over the abdomen and the organs which lie within it, including the uterus, a subject which deserves to be treated in more detail, and which we shall examine further in the next few pages.

THE DIAPHRAGM

The diaphragm is attached to the inside of the lower ribs, rather like an upside-down umbrella. Immediately above it and inside the cage of the thorax are the bottle-shaped lungs. As one breathes in, the diaphragm falls, flattens itself and spreads out, at the same time rising slightly at the edges, and the ribs are lifted by the intercostal muscles and spread out. It is a bit as if the umbrella were opened up, and since the outer spokes are attached to the ribs this causes the rib-cage to expand.

1. See Flanders Dunbar, *Emotions and Bodily Changes,* Columbia University Press, 1946.

Thus extra space is created in the thorax and one can fill the lungs with fresh air. When one breathes out again, the diaphragm relaxes and stale air is released, but there is always some residual air left in the lungs. When one has exhaled naturally and without strain, extra air can then be exhaled by using the muscles of the abdomen which are also attached to the lower ribs. As one exerts a strong pull on the abdominal muscles by pressing them in, the lungs are compressed so that carbon dioxide is forced out. The abdominal muscles used in this way terminate the respiratory activity which has been begun by the diaphragm.

From the sixth to seventh months of pregnancy the fundus of the uterus is much nearer the diaphragm, and each time the woman breathes in, the diaphragm is pressed down towards it. This can make breathing rather difficult until the time when the baby 'drops' or 'lightens' and there is more space around the middle. The obstetric term for this is *engagement* and it usually occurs any time after about six weeks before the baby is due in a woman having her first baby – but often not till nearer the expected date of confinement with a woman having her second or subsequent babies.

THE ABDOMINAL MUSCLES

The abdominal muscles are not consciously used in normal relaxed breathing. This happens only with powerful deep breathing such as may be used in voice production, in verse speaking, drama and singing. They do not need to be used consciously in labour either, and if they are, this may, I believe, actually hamper the woman in labour. The pressure of the abdominal muscles on the contracting uterus at the height of the first stage can be very uncomfortable, since it is acutely sensitive to pressure.

At first sight it would seem strange that the tightening of the abdominal wall could cause pain, and, indeed, some authorities believe this is unlikely. The movement of the abdominal wall in respiration is so obviously less drastic in its effects than the great waves of contraction undergone by the uterus. But the acute sensitivity of the uterus and surrounding layers of abdominal muscle to pressure during labour can be experienced during an otherwise painless contraction by simply strongly tensing the abdominal muscles at the height of the uterine contraction, as any woman in labour who is interested in the experiment can try. Women usually find *palpation* of the uterus (feeling, through the abdominal wall, the position in which the baby is lying) during a contraction also very painful, and midwives should try to avoid this. It used to be suggested by some of the first exponents of 'natural' or prepared methods of childbirth in Britain, notably Kathleen Vaughan[1] and Minnie Randall,[2] that steady pressure of the abdominal muscles during a contraction would speed up and ease the pains of labour by guiding the baby's head down into the pelvis and the birth canal. Those mothers who tried it may have experienced unnecessary pain.

The success which is claimed for the 'decompression suit', now on trial in various centres in Britain, would also seem to indicate that the contracting uterus is highly sensitive to any sort of pressure and that release of the abdominal muscles is contributory towards an easier labour. The mother lies in a plastic suit inside which, over the abdomen, is a fibre-glass dome. Attached to the suit is a vacuum pump, like an ordinary vacuum cleaner, to suck air out, and a pressure gauge. The decompression suit is said to go a long way towards relieving pain in the first stage of labour by applying extra-abdominal negative pressure to the contracting uterus, so drawing the abdominal wall forwards artificially and allowing the uterus to expand into a spherical shape at the height of the contractions.[3]

It has long been thought by some authorities – particularly the obstetric physiotherapists who followed Helen Heardman's teachings – that a tense abdominal wall would cause pain by pressure on the uterus, and relaxation was taught to avoid this, and also the specifically abdominal type of breathing which

1. Kathleen Vaughan, *Safe Childbirth*, Baillière, 1937.
2. Minnie Randall, *Training for Childbirth*, Churchill, 1949.
3. D. B. Scott and J. D. O. Loudon, 'A Method of Abdominal Decompression in Labour', *Lancet*, 28 May 1960.

usually took the form of teaching patients to breathe slowly in for fifteen seconds and slowly out for fifteen seconds, allowing the abdominal wall to expand with inhalation and to sink back with exhalation. This type of breathing had varying degrees of success, largely dependent upon whether or not the labouring woman was in fact able to move her abdominal wall at all once the first stage was well under way – since a good many women find this impossible (and I have not myself found this feasible). Moreover, if the respiratory movements are done jerkily and are not harmonized with contractions their value is completely lost and pain can result. An additional problem which this type of breathing may present is that women naturally want to breathe more rapidly during late first-stage contractions, and some conflict and stress can result from the endeavour to breathe very slowly.

The answer, I believe, is that the abdominal muscles can be released from tension and the pain of labour thereby reduced or even wiped out by *releasing the abdominal wall completely* – that is, by allowing it to rest, and by carefully avoiding, on the one hand, trying to keep it still (as has been recommended by some authorities), and, on the other, forcible movement of the abdominal wall when breathing in and out (which is recommended by other authorities) – both of which, in my experience, can lead to excessive pain.

The woman at the height of the first stage of labour should do shallow rapid breathing with the diaphragm raised and the abdominal muscles completely relaxed. Once she reaches two-thirds dilatation – usually once contractions are coming at about two – or three-minute intervals or less, or when contractions are experienced as being fierce and difficult to control – it may interest the woman who feels no fear of the experiment to shift from the shallow rapid breathing to slow deep abdominal breathing, forcing the abdominal wall out as she inhales.

RELAXATION OF THE ABDOMINAL MUSCLES

Some women find relaxation of the abdominal wall difficult, and especially so when they are experiencing any pain. They have been taught to 'hold their tummies in', and sometimes it runs against the grain to release these muscles. If a woman finds it does not come easily she must first make herself more aware of what contraction of these muscles feels like; only by doing the opposite to relaxation and by studying the movements associated with contraction of these muscles will she be able to learn how to let them 'give'.

This you will already have taught yourself to do when practising relaxation. Before you start the breathing exercises it is a good idea to do the girdle exercise again (Exercise 4, page 92 above) and concentrate attention on the abdominal muscles. Lie down on your back on the floor or a firm bed, a low pillow under the head and another under the knees, and relax. Do the girdle exercise, and then relax completely. Feel as if the tension has been 'peeled off' from the muscles.

In the same position, rest your fingers on your abdomen and lift your head to look at your toes. Immediately you will feel the pull of these abdominal muscles. Lie flat again and stretch right down one side; you will feel the pull of the lower abdominal muscles and all the muscles along that side of the abdomen. Now do the same with the other leg. Then bend your knees and relax, letting the abdominal wall go.

Now imagine that you are blowing on a candle flame about twelve inches in front of your pursed lips. You must bend the flame only, and blow on it with steady pressure without putting it out. In order to get the added control required for this you will find that you are automatically using the pressure of the abdominal muscles. You will feel them pulling just below the ribs, across the waistline and spreading out.

Once you are sure of the action of the abdominal muscles as you do these exercises, start to study the more subtle action of the diaphragm. One way of observing the action of the diaphragm is to breathe in fully and then breathe out in short, sharp rapid breaths as if you were panting after running fast. You will feel the diaphragm moving as you do this. Then close your lips, and make the diaphragm move in the same way without actually doing the panting breathing. When you do the candle-flame exercise, as you breathe in to blow the candle flame, the diaphragm drops slightly. It thins out and presses on the abdominal contents, and – if your baby is sufficiently high – also on the place where your baby's buttocks are. You will feel the pressure inside and slightly towards the back; as you continue to breathe in, the sensation spreads out sideways towards the ribs.

In the same way if you take a deep breath, feeling the diaphragm thinning out and pressing down as you do so, and then suddenly shout: 'Oh!' you will feel it spring back into position very rapidly.

THE TYPES OF BREATHING

1. *Slow breathing 'all down the back'*. This you have already learned when you were practising relaxation. Turn back to page 89 and practise this. It is useful if you feel over-excited at the start of labour, and also in between contractions in order to gain calm control of yourself and ensure that you are relaxed before the start of the next contraction.

2. *Slow full chest breathing*. This is used as soon as the contractions make the abdominal wall rigid, when you feel that you need to do something about meeting them. To practise, rest your hands at the sides of the ribs, spreading the fingers out so that you can feel as much of the bony cage as possible. Fill the lungs with air right down to the bottom, and you will feel the ribs swing out and up with each breath in, and swing down again with each breath out. These contractions last between thirty and fifty seconds, and the cervix is usually one to two or three fingers dilated. The interval between contractions is anything from about seven to about ten minutes. Once you have mastered this type of breathing you will not need to have your hands on the ribs. Relax them by your sides.

3. *Quicker, shallow chest breathing*. Now practise doing this more rapidly, when you will find that it is easier to use only the upper part of the chest, and possibly to breathe through the mouth in

order to get the air more quickly. As the contractions get more powerful you will find this more comfortable, as it will leave the lower part of the body to get on with the work of pulling open the cervix. In practice one does not need to adapt oneself immediately by going straight into this shallow breathing for

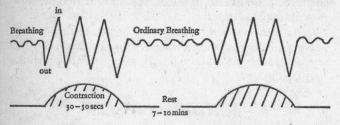

DEEP CHEST BREATHING: EARLY FIRST STAGE

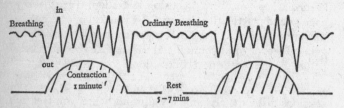

SHALLOW CHEST BREATHING: MIDDLE FIRST STAGE

Types of respiration for labour. The number of breaths to each contraction is unimportant: each woman will know what is best for her.

every contraction. One begins by taking a few slow breaths and as the contraction begins to mount to its height the breathing becomes more rapid and lighter. It then slows down again and becomes deeper as the contraction fades. The height of a contraction is about half or two-thirds of the way through, and it is then that one should be breathing most quickly and lightly. Finish each contraction with a long breath out, and rest. These contractions last about one minute and the cervix is usually two or three fingers dilated, or a little more. The interval between contractions is anything from about three-and-a-half to about seven minutes.

4. *Mouth-centred breathing* (shallow, rapid breathing). This is used at the end of the first stage, and is the shallowest and quickest type of breathing that you will be required to use. To practise, relax the shoulders and neck muscles, drop the jaw and breathe in and out through the mouth. Start slowly at first or you may find yourself gasping. It should be rhythmic and easy. Concentrate on sensations in the mouth rather than in the

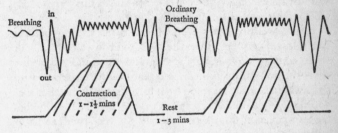

MOUTH-CENTRED BREATHING: LATE FIRST STAGE

In the *transition phase*, add to this a technique of blowing out. When the urge to push is great (at the height of the contraction) blow out hard, and continue with shallow rapid breathing without pausing.

throat or you may feel the air is 'catching' in the throat and you may cough. The head should be inclined slightly forward and the body relaxed. You may notice that your whole body seems to shake slightly; it is bound to do so if you are relaxed.

If you find this difficult – and it is one of the more difficult kinds of breathing to learn – think of a train in the distance; start very slowly and speed up as you get the knack of it. It is important to keep this breathing free and unstrained. Sometimes in classes we find it helpful to practise with a blown-up balloon on a string. The woman hangs the balloon just in front of her lips and breathes so that she feels she is 'patting' it very lightly with her breath.

Late first-stage contractions last about one minute, and occasionally as long as two minutes, and the interval between them is usually anything from about one minute to about three minutes, although sometimes two come almost on top of one another. Start the contraction slowly by breathing in and out deeply; then in again; drop the jaw and commence with the shallow chest breathing as you 'feel' for the rhythm of the contraction. As it begins to mount to its climax, centre the breathing in your mouth and speed up, till you reach the crest of the wave. Then the breathing begins to drop down, becoming slower and softer, till at the end of the contraction it fades away. Breathe out through your mouth, letting out as much stale air for as long as you can. Do not forget this, or you may feel breathless when doing this shallow breathing.

It is as well to rehearse this often, as the shallow quicker breathing is very helpful at the most difficult stage of labour when contractions are very strong and when there is a very short interval between them, and you need great self control and awareness of what to do to help yourself. Remember that your body must be relaxed and at peace. If your breathing becomes uneven at this stage you may get very tired, and this will mean not only that you are not on top of your form for the active second stage, but that you will feel pain much more easily. This type of breathing will see you through to four fingers dilatation.

A word of caution is, however, necessary here. The pace and depth of the breathing is a matter of very subtle adjustment according to the intensity and duration of the contractions. Only the woman in labour herself can judge the exact speed of respiration which helps her at that time. We have seen that some women tend to 'over-breathe' – tackling the whole process so energetically and enthusiastically that they breathe at once too deeply and too quickly, and this may result in an excessive loss of carbon dioxide from the lungs. It is most likely to happen if the woman gets into a state of panic, and this over-breathing is largely an *emotional* problem. Whoever is helping the labouring woman should remind her to breathe much more lightly, and can breathe with her over difficult contractions. A certain amount of carbon dioxide is usually residual in the lungs and acts as the normal stimulus to respiration. When this is flushed out a feeling of giddiness, pins and needles in the fingers and even cramp results. If these signs are noticed the respiratory response should be more relaxed and adjustment sought in a shallower, less vigorous type of breathing, and the breath can be held occasionally *in between* contractions. There are certain women who cope with their labours so intensely and with such deliberation of purpose that they over-play their role in this way. But it is important both in pregnancy and labour that women should experiment to find the right breathing *for them*. This is why I never speak of 'panting' breathing. It is *not* like a dog panting heavily on a hot summer's day or, if it is, more like a Pekinese than an Alsatian! When I was teaching this breathing to Jamaican women I found they soon learned it if I spoke of 'humming-bird breathing' and told them that it was as quick and light as the wings of a humming-bird fluttering up and down. Those readers who have seen humming-birds will be able to visualize this to help them.

If at any time you find that you lose the rhythm or feel as if the breath is getting caught in the throat, blow out quickly, and carry straight on. This can be practised using the balloon mentioned previously. Breathe lightly, and at every fifth or sixth breath, for example, blow out to blow the balloon away.

Simulating Contractions

If you and your husband can work together occasionally when practising, labour can be more or less 'rehearsed', and this can be particularly useful when learning how to adapt the different levels and rhythms of breathing to first-stage contractions.

It is important that you should learn how to relate yourself to tactile rather than purely verbal stimuli. In becoming more aware of muscle contractions in general you will be helped towards this, but it is often difficult or impossible to relate the types of breathing you have learned to muscle contractions which you deliberately perform in various parts of your body – a conscious and voluntary action which bears little or no relation to the involuntary activity of the uterus – or to spasmodic and brief Braxton-Hicks contractions. It is necessary to create something more in the nature of a true rehearsal of labour.

A method I have found very successful is to ask your husband to make a contraction for you by gradually tightening his hand over one of your legs and then releasing it, timing this process so that he starts with easy contractions lasting about half a minute and then increases the length and the manual pressure until you are having contractions of maximum intensity lasting one minute or more. He increases pressure up to the crest of each one, half or two-thirds of the way through. I have chosen to use pressure on one of the adductors since the nerve supply to the adductors is the same as that to the perineum, and the woman is involved in active release of those muscles directly associated with childbirth. The work a husband and wife can do together in this way, and the understanding he gets of labour contractions, is invaluable in their relationship and enables him to be sensitively aware of her needs during labour. Sometimes he makes two contractions very close together, or he makes a very steep crescendo to a contraction so that he can test her ability to adjust herself rapidly.

Women who have previously found shallow rapid breathing very difficult are often surprised to find how easily they adapt themselves to it given a 'real' contraction of this kind.

5. *Transition breathing*. The transition is the bridge between the first and second stages and once at this point you are well advanced in labour. The urge to press down on the baby to push it out may begin to establish itself, and is first felt as a *catch in the throat*. Mouth-centred breathing is also used through the transition phase, which may last only a few contractions, and may not occur at all (some women go straight from the first to the second stage) – the only variation being that it is often necessary to punctuate it by blowing out hard through pursed lips, rather more strongly than with the balloon blow, to prevent yourself bearing down as the contraction reaches its height and the urge to bear down is great. The rhythm of contractions has often changed by this time, and the climax of the contraction may come at the very end instead of somewhere in the middle, and, with this climax, the urge to

bear down. Then it is that you give a crisp, firm blow out similar to the sort of blow you would give if you were drinking lemonade through a straw and some of the lemon flesh got stuck in it. Practise doing three to six mouth-centred breaths and follow this by a quick blow and then continue immediately with the mouth-centred breathing, blow again, and so on, establishing a steady rhythm. This is an efficient method of stopping yourself pushing until the cervix is fully dilated and the way is clear for the baby to descend. Contractions often become very irregular in type and duration, and the interval between them varies during this phase.

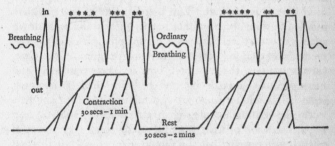

* While holding breath, allow yourself to bear down, relaxing and opening up below as you do so.

BREATHING FOR EXPULSION

These contractions are often irregular and uneven in intensity.

6. *Breathing for bearing down.* This is used for the expulsion of the baby in the second stage. To practise, breathe in, blow out; then take a deep breath in through the mouth, fixing the ribs and diaphragm, and, holding your breath, with your chin tucked in against your chest, and arms relaxed by your side and slightly flexed at the elbows, lean on the cushion of intra-abdominal pressure you can feel beneath the diaphragm and press down firmly and slightly outwards, feeling the muscles which will help you to squeeze your baby gently and evenly down the birth canal, at the same time deliberately *releasing the muscles of the pelvic floor*. It may help you to think of a tube of toothpaste which you are rolling up from the end with

steady pressure. Avoid all erratic straining and check that you are using only those muscles which are necessary to the action. In this type of breathing all pressure is from *above*, the diaphragmatic muscles helping the contracting uterus to press the baby down. There is no need to pull with your hands unless you have to lie flat, without pillows or other support behind your back; that is a waste of muscular effort and will tend to make you tighten up. Nor is there need to pull in the abdominal muscles to perform this action; they should be released. You will observe the pressure pass right down through the abdomen until you feel it on the pelvic floor and you feel the vulva open wide.

In labour, if the contraction is still powerful and you have finished pushing, take another breath quickly and press down again. You may feel the baby's head slipping back at the end of the contraction, but it is making progress every time. Contractions of the expulsive type last between thirty and forty seconds and the interval between them is anything from half a minute to about two minutes. As the baby gets lower the contractions may change their nature and you may get a succession of weak ones following some very powerful ones. It is important that you should adapt yourself to this and press down only as firmly as the contractions indicate. You may also notice that you get an occasional longer interval for rest between contractions, and should take full advantage of this to relax completely and breathe deeply.

Sometimes the baby is coming very fast and feels as if it is surging out; this is very likely to be the case with second and subsequent babies, and occurs sometimes with first babies too. It is unnecessary to push hard in these cases, and the mother can best help the birth and avoid excessive strain on the perineum if, after doing a couple of deep breaths in and out at the start of each contraction, she moves straight up into mouth-centred breathing, and then holds her breath only when she absolutely must, and when the urge to do so is passionate and imperative. The sensation is something she can be in no two minds about, any more than she would about reaching the orgasmic peak when she was making love. As soon as she can breathe rapidly and lightly again, she does so, holding her breath again only when the urge is overwhelming, and so on. As the contraction passes she moves 'down the slope' into slow breathing, does a long breath out, and relaxes completely till the next contraction. As a general rule, I find that once an area of the baby's head can be seen about the size of an after-dinner coffee cup in the vagina it is usually best to do this type of breathing and holding, rather than to continue with deep breathing. The use of a delivery mirror is especially useful at this point to enable the mother to realize when this stage has been reached. But this is very much a matter of co-operation between the woman and the person delivering her, and she should at all times follow the instructions of her attendant, although frequently there is ample opportunity between contractions for questions and discussions.

It is a good idea to do these exercises twice a day when practising relaxation, but if this is impossible, try to get to bed a little earlier and to run through them before you go to sleep. The last exercise should be practised only once a week unless you choose to rehearse it when you are on the lavatory. It is an effective remedy for constipation.

It is important to emphasize again that only the mother herself can tell when it is best to use each type of breathing. She should practise all kinds. However, if contractions start coming at intervals of less than five minutes and are powerful she may find it helps to start mouth-centred breathing immediately labour starts. In the case of precipitate births in which labour lasts under five hours, rapid adjustment is necessary, and a quick evaluation of the nature of the contractions and the correct respiratory response to them.

Learning the different levels and rates of breathing for labour is, however, a *rudimentary exercise*, a little as one might learn scales before proceeding to play music on the piano. The actual finger exercises are not those required for labour, and only give the basic technical equipment, which must then be built into the 'music' with which the breathing relates to contractions. This may be most easily conceptualized, after the initial few practice sessions, by thinking in terms not of exercises at all, but of 'wave breathing'.

WAVE BREATHING

As the wave of the contraction rises, the breathing adjusts by becoming shallower and more rapid, and the woman lifts her breathing up and over the contraction like a hovercraft on the water. We have seen that contractions come as waves of pressure at varying but steadily decreasing intervals in an undulating, rhythmic pattern, and that the height of the contraction is like the crest of the wave. And, as with waves of the sea, each one contributes to the sweep forward of the incoming tide, which is the birth of the baby. This feeling of rhythmic flow, or a natural sweep of events, helps the woman in labour to integrate initially isolated techniques into a total pattern of psychosomatic adjustment – and it is this total pattern which is all-important.

It is helpful if the woman always listens to the sound of her breathing, so that her conscious appreciation of its rhythm prevents any possibility of it 'running away' with her. If at any point she loses the rhythm, tensing her throat muscles, or has the impression that her breath is being 'caught', she merely blows out crisply as if blowing a balloon away from her, and carries straight on. Never continue mouth-centred breathing desperately if you feel uncomfortable, but simply blow in this way, and this blow out can then find a place within your breathing patterns as you proceed through the late first stage and into the second.

To keep the breathing comfortable, light and effortless, the muscles of the face, mouth and neck should be relaxed. Once a woman's head is pressed back into the pillow, her face fixed like a mask, or her chin thrown up in the air, muscle tensions are involved which may build up until she is panting heavily. So breathing for labour cannot be divorced from the study of relaxation. Lightness can be maintained by thinking in terms of an image – 'like a bubble on top of a wave', 'a sparrow's feather', 'a butterfly's wings', 'a humming-bird drawing nectar

from a flower', 'tissue paper in the breeze', 'a leaf on a birch
tree', 'a balloon hanging by an open window, patted against
the wall by a breath of wind', or any other suitable image.

PRACTISING BREATHING WITH BRAXTON-HICKS CONTRACTIONS

Contractions of the uterus occur not only in labour but
throughout pregnancy. Before labour starts the 'trial' contractions are known as Braxton-Hicks contractions. A woman
is unlikely to notice these until the later months of pregnancy.
First, she may think it is her baby moving, but she will
notice if she lays a hand on her abdomen that it is hard, pro-
tuberant and firm, and that as the movement dies down the
abdominal wall becomes relatively soft again. It feels a little
as if the baby were turning a somersault, but at the point when
he has half turned he stays rigid and immobile for some seconds. That is the height of the contraction, and sometimes it
is so strong and feels so surprising that she will find herself
holding her breath. If a woman gets recognizable Braxton-
Hicks contractions it is a good idea also to practise breathing
for labour sometimes when they occur, as this prepares her for
harmonizing respiration and the rhythm of the contraction.
These contractions are of the same nature as those experienced
in labour, but when labour starts they recur at regular intervals.

If you get the opportunity to relax while watching trees
swaying in a storm, this can also provide an occasion for
practising adapting yourself to a rhythm which is somewhat
like that of labour. Lie or sit and check that you have complete
muscular release. Keeping your eyes on the branches in the
wind feel your relaxed body adjust itself to the sweep of the
storm, and you will discover that your breathing rhythm has
altered and is following the movement of the biggest branches
as they are driven in a wide arc by the wind. The branches do
not crack because they go with the wind and do not resist it.
They bend and give with the storm in much the same way as
you will find harmony in your labour.

SECOND STAGE CO-ORDINATION

Bearing down

It is commonly supposed that the abdominal muscles need to be used forcefully in expulsive effort during the second stage of labour. In classes for preparation for childbirth, women are often taught how to use these muscles and to press the abdominal wall in on to the contracting uterus. They are taught how to relax them for the first stage of labour, but are expected to be able to contract them for the second stage. This however is not only unnecessary but undesirable. The action by which the baby is pressed down the birth canal should be piston-like, with all pressure being exerted from above on to the fundus of the uterus, and the pelvic floor muscles completely relaxed. If you hold a cardboard cylinder in your hand and press a marble through it from the top (with a finger of the other hand performing the role of the diaphragm) the journey will be made rather more difficult if you grip the cylinder firmly than if you release the pressure.

If the abdominal wall is drawn taut and pressed in on to the contracting uterus, pressure is necessarily exerted on the sides of the uterus and in this way the pressure from above is prevented from having its full effect.

Think of your uterus as a mammoth pear or ripe fig, the stalk of which lies below the diaphragm at the mid-point of the abdomen and which is tilted down towards the buttocks. Take a deep breath in, fix the ribs and the diaphragm and, holding your breath, feel as if you are pressing down from the stalk end right through the whole pear shape till you reach the very bottom of it. It will help to feel as if you are leaning on a bolster of air in the abdomen. If you place your cupped hands at the bottom of the abdomen, just where you begin to curve in again, you will feel your muscles pushing your hands down and out away from your body.[1] You should press right down

1. Some women find it easiest to think of a pyramid, the base of which is formed by the big hip-bones and the top of which is formed by the centre of the diaphragm. They exert pressure from that point right down through to the base at its widest.

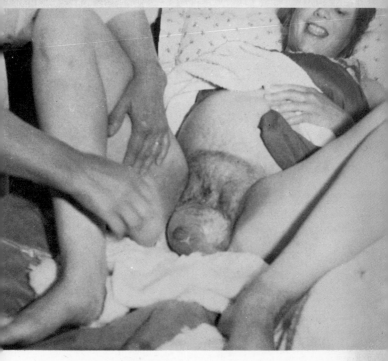

The second stage of labour. The mother has not been shaved in this case. Relaxed and laughing, with mouth open, she 'breathes out' the baby's head. The top of the baby's head, egg-shaped, and with the glint of the membranes still visible on the crown, is slowly slipping out.

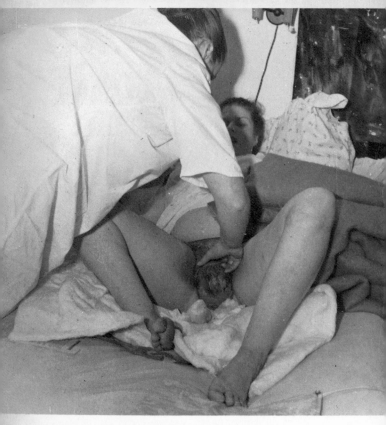

The midwife feels to find out if the cord is around the baby's neck. The baby here is facing down towards the bed.

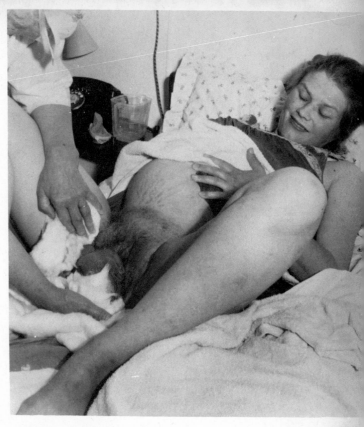

The mother looks down at her baby's face. The head rotates from left to right. (The bump above is the second twin, still inside.)

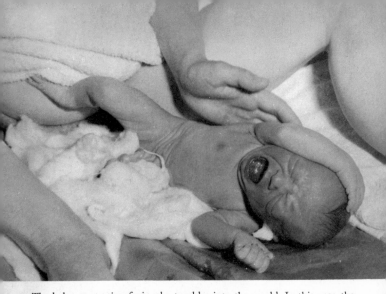

The baby, protesting furiously, tumbles into the world. In this case the mother's own hands deliver the baby's body.

The midwife waits for the cord to stop pulsating before tying and cutting it.

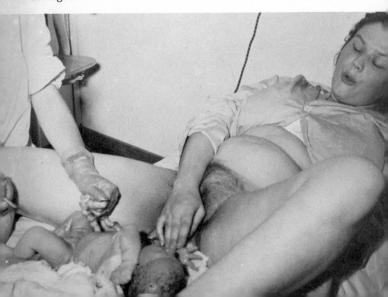

from the diaphragm until you feel the movement on the pelvic floor and the vagina will automatically open up.

Now do the opposite movement, pressing the abdominal wall in hard. You will see that it is much more difficult to relax the muscles of the birth outlet at the same time, and that the movement is in itself rather uncomfortable, making you feel as if you are being laced into a corset that is much too tight. The baby will still be born if you use this movement, but the untaught woman who is unafraid and fully conscious will spontaneously use the previous movement rather than this one, and she is right in her instinctive response to the message coming from her uterus.

To practise bearing down in this way, lie on a bed or couch well supported with pillows with your husband sitting on your left side with his arm around you. See that the lower part of the spine – the sacrum and coccyx – is lying flat on the surface of the bed.

Breathing for the crowning[2]

After you have practised the bearing-down movement as described above once or twice your husband should suddenly interrupt your efforts with the command 'Stop pushing', and you should instantly stop and start panting lightly so that the baby's head can be delivered more slowly as you 'breathe it out'. Your husband should give you no warning of when he is going to say this, and you should rehearse this technique until the response is perfect.

2. The point at which the top of the baby's head protrudes and does not slip back again.

CHAPTER 6

Learning Harmony in Labour: Relaxing the Birth Outlet

WE have seen already that it is important to know how to exercise the muscles of the pelvic floor, how to release them while the baby is being born, and how to keep them firmly tensed in the weeks following the baby's birth so the rehabilitation is complete. Now I shall describe how one can learn to isolate and control these muscles so that they can be released and contracted at will and their tone increased. These are some of the most important exercises a woman can do, *whether pregnant or not*. Look back first at the diagrams on page 43.

Exercise 1

Pull in all the muscles between the legs, *without tensing the thighs or buttocks*. Pull them right in, draw them up as strongly as you can, and hold it. Then release them so that they are quite soft and seem to be falling away from you, like a hammock, from the large bones of the pelvis. As they are released it may help you to think of a lift going right down to the bottom floor of a high building. Check that you release the muscles completely and do not stop three-quarters of the way down. Now release them that little bit more. Now pull in again, letting the lift ascend, first, second, third, fourth, fifth, sixth floor, and hold it there. Relax. Finally pull in and hold.

Exercise 2

Draw in and tighten the very powerful sphincter of the anus (back passage) without tensing the muscles around the vagina directly. Do this very gently and slowly. Since the *levator ani*, although composed of different muscular segments, stretches right across the perineum, it is impossible to isolate each completely, but experiment to see how delicate a muscular control you can achieve. Then deliberately release the muscles. Finish by pulling in again.

Exercise 3

Now feel as if you are constricting a ring of muscle about half-way up inside the vagina. Most of the tightening should be at the front and you should feel only a slight ripple of muscular contraction towards the anus. You feel the ring tighten to an oval, and get narrower and tighter still, till you feel as if you could hold a hazel-nut inside with the muscles. You feel the top circle of something like a figure-of-eight of muscle fibres tightening, and at the same time the transverse perineal muscle stretching across at the crossing point of the figure-of-eight is drawn forward towards the pubis. Then release the muscles. Finally pull them in.

For most women the feeling is familiar, as this is 'a kiss inside' when making love, but some are very frightened of using these muscles, or use them only involuntarily, in spasm, because they hate the idea of intercourse or of being examined vaginally by a doctor. This exercise will help you to gain conscious control over the muscles, so that you can do exactly what you like with them, contract or release them, just as you wish. Sometimes gaining increased awareness of these muscles can be a great help in a marriage.

Exercise 4

There is an even deeper level of muscle up inside the front passage, rather nearer the bladder. Now pull in the ring of muscle you have just been exercising, and then draw in and up the muscles just underneath the pubis, at about the level of the hair-line. If you rest your fingers there you will be able to feel them working deep inside. These muscles help to support the bladder. Relax. Contract.

Exercise 5

Once you have achieved this delicate control, practise tightening the buttock muscles (the glutei) without contracting the pelvic floor muscles. Imagine that you have a £5 note between your buttocks and someone is trying to take it away from you. Relax. Tighten the buttock muscles again, and then pull in the pelvic floor and hold both contractions. Still holding the buttock muscles tight, relax the pelvic floor. Relax completely. Now contract the buttock muscles again, then the pelvic floor as well; then slowly and steadily release the buttocks – let them open out away from each other while keeping the pelvic floor tight. Difficult, but it comes with practice.

Exercise 6

Now press the tops of the legs towards each other, tightening the adductors, without contracting the pelvic floor muscles. Relax and let the legs flop apart. Now tighten the tops of your legs again, and then pull in the pelvic floor and hold both contractions. Still holding the adductors tight, relax the pelvic floor. Relax completely. Now contract the adductors again, then the pelvic floor as well; release the adductors while keeping the pelvic floor tight. Relax completely.

You will see that you do not need to contract either buttock muscles or muscles in your legs to contract the pelvic floor. Pelvic floor exercises are, therefore, invisible ones, and can be done anywhere, standing waiting to be served in a shop, at a cocktail party, waiting for a bus, or washing up, and as you get more adept you will not even show on your face that you are concentrating on exercises. It is a good idea to do them whenever you feel rather weary, when you have to stand for any length of time, and when you go up or down stairs.

Exercise 7

There are muscles further at the back of the pelvic floor, just where your tail would be if you had one. Babies often have a deep dimple there. Feel to the bottom of your spine, where the division in your buttocks begins. See if you can 'wag the tail up'. Move your fingers until you find the place where the movement is coming from. Relax. See if you can wag the tail up and down, up and down. Now do it from side to side – more difficult – and you will find it easier if you move your lips at the same time. Now relax completely. Contract the whole pelvic floor and maintain good tone.

These muscles sometimes contract when the labouring woman does not like the feeling of the baby's head pressing against her lower back, right at the bottom of her spine, as it journeys lower, and often she starts lifting her buttocks up off the bed at the same time. Now you have learned how to release them deliberately, so helping the baby's head down and forward.

This delicate muscular coordination does not come easily at first and requires much practice. When you have an internal examination at some time during your pregnancy you can check with your doctor to find out if you are doing this properly. It is easy to feel when you are gripping the examining finger or when you are pushing it out, but you may need help in achieving complete muscular release there. If you practise stopping the stream of urine occasionally when you are emptying your bladder you will gain added control over the pelvic floor muscles.

When your baby's head is being born you will have to release all these muscles or you may be torn or may require an episiotomy (a cut), and whilst you hardly feel that at the time, it can be uncomfortable afterwards for some days or weeks. When the baby's head is actually pressing against the perineum you can discuss this with your doctor or midwife, and ask whether the perineum seems to be soft and stretchy enough; if they appear doubtful, ask whether you may 'blow away' a few contractions so that the birth takes place more gently and the tissues get time to fan out. Sometimes, of course, it is important to get the baby delivered as soon as possible, and this is not a good idea. Older mothers are less likely to have elastic tissues here, and an episiotomy may help them.

ASSOCIATION BETWEEN MOUTH AND VAGINA

Yet we face a problem here, in that when one wants anything too much and concentrates one's thoughts upon it to the exclusion of all else, the very opposite may result. This is particularly true with relaxation of any part of the body. When the baby's head, feeling very large indeed, is pressing solidly against the pelvic floor, it is easy to tense up those muscles even when the mother is trying to release them.

Muscular release can be greatly helped at this point by having established and trained oneself during the later months of pregnancy in a system of conscious association between the part of the body which is under stress and another part which is not under stress.

There is a strange unconscious neuro-muscular association between the vagina and the mouth. The pads of flesh at either side of the vagina are even called *labia* (lips). Our earliest experiences of erotic delight are centred in our mouths and lips and associated with pleasurable feeding. Even when our eroticism has developed to full genital maturity we retain a pleasure in stimulation of the surfaces of the lips and tongue, which are still sensitive to touch: we enjoy kissing; some smoke; others chew gum or sweets or chocolates. We never entirely outgrow our early infantile mouth-centredness.

When a woman proves tense in the region of the pelvic floor she can often be helped to relax by teaching her how to relax her mouth and jaw. If one then asks her to get the same feeling of looseness in the area of the vagina she can do it with far less difficulty. But if she starts tightening up her mouth, she finds that she is automatically tightening up the pelvic floor too.

In photographs of deliveries of mothers who had no laceration it is remarkable that the mother has her mouth open as the head is crowning and being born. She is smiling or laughing and her lips are parted in pleasure and anticipation. In old-fashioned midwifery it was sometimes customary for the midwife to instruct the mother to open her mouth and scream or shout as the baby's head started to bulge through the perineum. This must have afforded a noticeable release of tension, since one cannot scream fully unless the jaw is dropped and the mouth wide open. Perhaps midwives were unconsciously using a technique the conscious use of which in a modified and more constructive form could be applied to modern natural childbirth.

To build up a conscious association between mouth and birth outlet, start by inclining your head forward and releasing the muscles of the lips, throat and tongue. The jaw should feel as if it is hanging from the cheek-bones and from just below the ears. If you put your finger-tips over those points and then let your jaw drop it may prove easier. Feel as if you are wearing very heavy ear-rings. See that the tip of your tongue is resting against the back of the lower front teeth and the lips are slightly parted. At the same time feel the soft palate spread wider apart and relaxed, opening out from the shape of a Gothic to a Roman arch. Now concentrate upon the area of the birth outlet

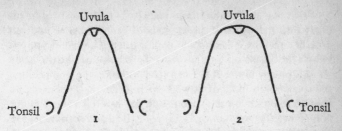

Diagrammatic representation of the movement of the soft palate as its muscles are released.

1. Here the palato-pharyngeal arch is contracted. This sort of contraction results when one feels as if an aspirin is stuck in the throat.
2. Here the palato-pharyngeal arch is relaxed.

and tense up all those muscles hard, and hold them back. Involuntarily you will discover that you have tightened muscles in your throat and that your jaw has become rigid and that you have either curled the tip of your tongue back or started to push it against the front teeth.

Now release the muscles of the mouth and pelvic floor and start again, but this time commence with the relaxation of the pelvic floor. Then relax your mouth. Now firmly clench your teeth, tighten your lips, throat and tongue. If the birth outlet is still relaxed you have quite extraordinary control. Now relax both mouth and pelvic floor. Keep them relaxed like this for a minute or so. Breathe in and out gently and slowly through your parted lips and at the same time feel as if you are 'breathing with the vagina'.

This is what you want your body to do when the baby's head is being pressed through the outlet. Imagine that you have the baby's head, much the size of a grapefruit, in the vulva, and help it to bulge forward by releasing the muscles in this way. Every time that you rehearse bearing down, and especially when rehearsing the panting breathing you can use when the head crowns and when you have suddenly to stop pushing, *relax your mouth* and let the jaw drop from the cheek-bones. Be particularly careful that when you pant you do not at the same time tense up your lips and throat. The head should be well tilted forward on to the chest.

When you are in labour and your baby is about to make his entry into the world it is extremely difficult to know yourself whether you are relaxing the birth outlet. The feeling of the baby's head is so unfamiliar that it hardly seems like the body you know any more. It is like a seed pod bursting open or like the speeded-up films of flowers opening in sunlight that one sees occasionally on television. But you can tell what you are doing with your mouth, and your husband can also see whether you are relaxing there. So as the baby approaches the perineum, gradually distends it and then slowly oozes through the birth outlet, concentrate upon relaxation of the lips, tongue and throat, and feel the muscles over your cheeks beginning to stretch. You will find no difficulty in this, and if you are leaning forward slightly so as to watch your baby's birth and to control it more delicately you will probably be smiling.

The inability to relax the muscles of the pelvic floor easily and spontaneously may be associated with deeply unconscious factors and particularly with the extent to which the individual has developed from the anal erotic stage to full genital eroticism. This hypothesis was presented by John Rickman, who suggested that when an individual failed to reach the point at which she could renounce infantile sexuality for someone outside herself weakness in the pelvic floor and of the ligaments which hold up the uterus might result.[1]

'In normal labour, for instance, during the second stage, the uterine contractions exert a force proportional to the resistance of the lower genital canal; the perineum is able to bear all the force instinctively exerted without injury ... but if the woman, from excitement or from pain, begins to use all her force to end the labour speedily we know that there is grave risk of laceration of the perineum.' John Rickman believed that there were psychological reasons why certain women gave way to excitement or pain in this way and behaved hysterically, taking 'the tempo of their voluntary exertions' neither from 'the rhythm of the uterine contractions nor from the bidding

1. 'A Psychological Factor in the Aetiology of Descensus Uteri, Laceration of the Perineum and Vaginismus', *Selected Contributions to Psycho-Analysis,* ed. W. Clifford, M. Scott, Hogarth Press, 1957.

of their obstetrician'. He saw it as panic in face of a pyscho-sexual situation in which the woman lost touch with the doctor, as she had previously with her husband in intercourse, and 'behaves regressively, expelling the child, as she expels faeces, with force and without delicacy'. Where the midwife takes the place of the male doctor the situation would, how-ever, appear to be rather different, but there probably still remains in the process of giving birth a sexual element of which women become dimly aware and which tends to fright-en some. Possibly a woman who has come to terms with the sexual side of her nature, and who is capable of a sexual gratification in which another person is involved, is better able to adjust herself to the genital stimulus with a unified, co-ordinated psycho – sexual response, to release the muscles of the pelvic floor and to bear down with delicacy and without un-necessary force.

At the conclusion of each session of pelvic floor exercises – and particularly when one has been rehearsing the sensations of helping the baby's head to 'bulge forward' – it is very im-portant to remember to contract the muscles gently but firmly, to hold them this way and to continue holding them firm. Just as we do not go around with eyelids drooping or jaw dropped, so the pelvic floor should not be slack, but should have good muscle tone. Awareness of these muscles leads to increased voluntary control over them, both in terms of ability to release them and in terms of maintenance of muscle tone.

CHAPTER 7

A Note to Husbands

'I thought the best husbands looked on their wives' lying-in as a time of festival and jollity. What! Did you not even get drunk in the time of your wife's delivery? Tell me honestly how you employed yourself at this time.'

'Why then honestly,' replied he, 'and in defiance of your laughter, I lay behind her bolster and supported her in my arms.'

HENRY FIELDING *Amelia*, first published in 1751.

THROUGHOUT this book I refer to the presence of the husband during labour; he is at the centre of the drama by his wife's side. He it is who rubs her back during the first stage; he regulates and corrects her breathing, sees that she is fully awake and concentrating on her task, and helps her to check that she is relaxed; and it is against him that she leans as she gives birth to the child. Perhaps he is the first person to see the baby and it may even be in his arms that it first falls asleep.

This is the right place for the husband to be. It is not only ludicrous but pathetic to leave him to stride up and down a hospital corridor, smoking cigarette after cigarette, whilst his wife 'gets on with it' alone. Nor is the situation greatly improved if he waits at the bottom of the stairs straining his ears to catch each sound issuing from the bedroom, feeling that his only function is to boil up ever more saucepans of water for the midwife.[1]

1. It is sometimes difficult for older doctors and midwives to appreciate the closeness that many young married couples have nowadays, and to understand that often the husband considers it really important to be at his wife's side during her labour. The doctor in his early forties who told a pregnant woman, 'I have never seen my wife in labour – never wanted to; always been downstairs, listening', failed to realize that for this couple the wife would have seen her husband's voluntary absence from the birth as a failure in love.

The last requirement of all for a successful delivery at home is the husband – the poor father. If he is of the right mentality, and very few are, he may sustain his wife's morale during the first part of her labour. Otherwise he is best employed making tea, keeping the kettles boiling, and answering the front door bell.

Thus is the father condescendingly referred to in a B.M.A. publication, *You and Your Baby*. We are not told how many pots of tea and how many kettles of water the father will have succeeded in boiling at the end of a sixteen-hour labour, nor what anyone is going to do with it all. As occupational therapy it is perhaps as good as anything, but it would appear both to be wasteful and to deny the woman in labour the reassurance, the active assistance and the loving care of her husband, who is, after all, the father of this child who is making his way into the world.

There is, in fact, no need for the husband to be a figure of fun and of music-hall jokes, who is treated as if he had neither the intelligence nor the humanity to be of any help. He can and should be the one person whom his wife feels she must have with her, her guide and counsellor, who will gently and firmly correct her faults, encourage her when she begins to lose confidence, and let her know by his pride in her that she is doing well.

Husbands who have experienced childbirth shared in this way, even when they had not previously intended to be present and stayed only because their wives wanted it very much, say nearly always one thing – 'It was wonderful.' In the words of one new father

'I can see why some husbands would not enjoy their wife's labour. But what they miss! The feeling that one can genuinely soothe, help and encourage one's wife and share the climax of birth seems to me to deepen the warmth and understanding of a marriage.'

On the other hand it is as well to remember that the husband who is present without having a clue as to how he can best help his wife may not only feel superfluous but may actually be in the way. With some previous study, however, he will have learned how to foresee his wife's wishes, and will already know approximately what to expect. Since he understands labour as a process of which the actual birth is the natural climax – not an isolated, traumatic and shocking occurrence – it is extremely unlikely that his child's arrival will cause him to faint, a reaction sometimes shown by husbands taken by surprise which, with justification, tends to prejudice certain midwives against the husband's presence. As one new father put it, 'I could never bear having an injection or the sight of blood. I'm squeamish about these things generally, but when a husband is there from the beginning and has a job to do – rubbing his wife's back and helping her with her breathing – then there is no shock involved. It all seems perfectly natural.'

In order to be of maximum assistance to his wife in labour, I would suggest that a man should do the following things:

DURING HIS WIFE'S PREGNANCY

Read some of the books on childbirth she is reading. Discuss them with her and help her to sort out any ideas or details of the methods described which seem obscure. In the chapters on pregnancy and the chapters on 'The Mother and Her Baby' and 'The Parents' Adjustment', in this book there are references to the marital relationship which may be useful. He should certainly look at the photographs in Pierre Vellay's *Childbirth Without Pain*[1] which give a much better impression visually of the sort of thing that will be going on during labour than I can give in words.

Go with his wife at least once when she visits her doctor to make arrangements for a labour in which she is given full opportunity to benefit from her preparation during pregnancy. If the midwife, rather than a doctor, is to be present at the confinement discuss these matters with her.

Make his wife feel desired and attractive.

Help his wife with her exercises, including her different types of breathing, and relaxation, and do some of them himself, so that he realizes what the difficulties are. A good time is when they get into bed at night. They need not make a

1. Hutchinson, 1959.

ritual of this, but should try to do it three or four times a week.

Stand between his wife and the sceptics, the bearers of old wives' tales and those who see birth as a sort of major surgical operation. Let her see that he has complete confidence in her and in her capacity to have her baby naturally.

DURING LABOUR

If at home, prepare the room. Pull the bed out if it is not already at right angles to the wall and help his wife make it up with old sheets and a rubber sheet underneath. (Many women like a painting or a bowl of flowers to concentrate on during contractions.)

Stay with his wife throughout labour.

Keep a log book of the labour, noting the timing and duration of contractions, and signs of progress.

Help her to keep calm and to keep her head. Remind her of the respiratory and muscular responses necessary. As the first stage progresses and each contraction comes he says, 'Breathe in – breathe out – ' to help her to steady herself as she meets it, or says, 'Begin controlled breathing', and may breathe with her.

Explain to the midwife or obstetrician what his wife is trying to do if they ask him. See that his wife is given no analgesia unless she agrees to it. The husband's task is not, of course, to *prevent* her accepting analgesics, but rather to see that they are not – as occasionally still happens – forced upon her if she herself feels she does not require them. It goes without saying that the husband should not use the special close relation he has with his wife to dissuade her from accepting help if she needs it, and he should be sufficiently perceptive to observe if his wife is putting up a bold front but really needs analgesia although she does not like to admit it.

Be ready with early contractions to massage her back firmly in the sacral area – near where the big hip-bones join the spine, or massage her hips and thighs if she has pain there.

Refresh and stimulate her with sips of fruit juice, water,

strong, sweet black coffee or other drinks if she wants them. Water only should be taken once contractions are coming regularly five minutes or less apart.

As the end of the first stage approaches, wring out sponges or flannels in very cold, preferably iced, water, and rest them against her forehead, the nape of her neck, and possibly also over her lips. An electric fan also may help if she is feeling very hot.

Give her extra blankets and hot water bottles if she feels shivery at the end of the first stage. She will probably appreciate a hot water bottle at her feet, and one tucked in the small of her back may help to relieve pain. If she finds it difficult to relax her legs one between the tops of the legs will probably help.

Give her barley sugar, or sugar, or anything sweet to suck if she wants it early in labour. This helps her keep up her energy.

Help her into the position for the second stage, leaning back against his arm.

Remind her to tilt her head forward on to her chest before she bears down for a contraction, and to open her mouth and relax the muscles of the cheek, neck and tongue as the baby's head is about to crown in order to facilitate relaxation of the pelvic floor.

AFTER DELIVERY

But all this is only the beginning. Once the child is born the wife should feel that however bad a mother she is, however she fails, however others criticize her, *he* believes in her.

He should also be quick to see how and when he can help his wife when he is at home. Husband and wife may be able to learn something from each other in their handling of the baby, and no husband need feel that just because she is a woman his wife is necessarily more skilled in baby management. When parenthood is a shared enterprise not only does it become more fun for both, but the children benefit from not being confined to the care of one person all the time.

Childbirth is not an illness, but work for which the female

body is efficiently and most exquisitely constructed. It should be a truly 'happy event' taking place in an atmosphere of tranquillity and loving care. Teams of skilled nurses, batteries of sterile instruments, rows of antiseptically clean and shining delivery rooms, and spotless nurseries shielded by plate glass cannot ensure that this atmosphere is created. But the friendly, nursing care of the midwife and the support of a husband who cherishes his wife and shares with her pleasure in the baby's birth – these in themselves take a woman a long way towards childbirth which brings with it exultant joy.

And the end of it all – the purpose for which there is all this organization and care – the baby. The new father greets his child:

As for the baby, I was frightened by it. Such frailty; the paper-thin, yet powerful, cry. A living being, warm and wet from the womb, utterly helpless, bemused, staring about with bright eyes. Tiny fingers and fingernails plucking at the air. Perhaps it is a sense of responsibility that frightens me, or some primeval feeling of guilt. I have helped to create a life; a pulsing being that might be crushed sooner or later in a million different ways: a small accident, an illness, in a cataclysm. Yet the baby having been born, one feels its journey is ended, not just begun. That it should suffer the risks of life seems unfair. Before this tiny presence those risks seem formidable. One is acutely aware of the preciousness of life. One drives with extra care this day. One sees people about one as more real people.[1]

Laurie Lee, in *The Firstborn*,[2] is stirred by the same helplessness:

She was born in the autumn and was a late fall in my life, and lay purple and dented like a little bruised plum, as though she'd been lightly trodden in the grass and forgotten.

Then the nurse lifted her up and she came suddenly alive, her bent legs kicking crabwise, and her first living gesture was a thin wringing of the hands accompanied by a far-out Hebridean lament.

1. From one father's account of the birth of his baby. See Sheila Kitzinger, *Giving Birth: the parents' emotions in childbirth,* Gollancz, 1971.
2. Hogarth Press, 1963.

This moment of meeting seemed to be a birthtime for both of us; her first and my second life. Nothing, I knew, would be the same again, and I think I was reasonably shaken. I peered intently at her, looking for familiar signs, but she was convulsed as an Aztec idol. Was this really my daughter, this purple concentration of anguish, this blind and protesting dwarf?

Then they handed her to me, stiff and howling, and I held her for the first time and kissed her, and she went still and quiet as though by instinctive guile, and I was utterly enslaved by her flattery of my powers.

CHAPTER 8

The Beginnings of Labour

He cam al so stylle,
There his moder was,
As dew in Aprille
That fallyt on the gras.
He came al so stylle
To his moderes bour,
As dew in Aprille
That fallyt on the flour.
He came al so stylle
There his moder lay,
As dew in Aprille
That fallyt on the spray.
Anonymous (early fifteenth century)

IN this chapter we are concerned with labour not merely as a physiological and mechanical process in which the patient is caught up, but with the woman as a *person* who is giving birth. The emphasis is not only upon the birth, but on the *giving* – on the woman's capacity to give herself to the creative process and the transmission of life. It is not only that a woman has a baby inside her which is ripe to be born: she longs to savour the experience of birth to the full, not wanting to hold back or to give only half of herself to the task, and she can learn how to express her joy in the birth through her body.

THE WOMAN'S ATTITUDE TO LABOUR

Three different influences seem to be at work to affect the nature of a woman's attitude to her labour.

Firstly, cultural factors determine a woman's acceptance of labour, her adjustment to it and the rituals which surround it. These cultural factors account for the *style* of childbirth in any given society. Grantly Dick-Read drew attention to culturally induced fear of the childbirth process current in our own society, in which stories relating to pain and endurance are handed down from mother to daughter and from older married women to young girls, stories which find a place in our literature and films and in the folk literature of the magazine romance.[1] Nicolaiev in the U.S.S.R. and Lamaze in France based their teaching upon the desirability of destroying the unpleasant associations thus conditioned by society and the subsequent re-education of the sympathetic nervous system. This is no simple task, for the cultural factors which they sought to neutralize also include the taboos which surround childbirth, the social sanctions which maintain and reinforce tradition, the roles and functions of doctors and midwives in our society, and the roles in which fathers and mothers are accepted in relation to their children. To understand childbirth in its institutionalized form one would have to know much about the structure of the society concerned and the relations between the groups of people within it.

The degree of medical knowledge and the way in which it is applied in the society also affect any individual woman's approach to her labour. The machinery which modern Western society puts into operation in any individual case is limited and modified by physiological facts of health or disease – facts relating to scientific medical knowledge concerning the size of the foetus in relation to the mother's pelvis, the presentation of the foetus, etc.

But over and above this we meet the woman's personality and her acceptance or rejection of the experiences with which life presents her and all the factors which compose this – the

1. This culturally induced fear ranges through the whole gamut of literary output, from light suggestion, epitomized by the heroine of the magazine romance whose labour pains are hinted at rather than described: '"I must relax, I *must* relax," she muttered fiercely'; to the full realistic treatment afforded by some films (though none the less sometimes inaccurate), as in the vivid scene – which I remember from my own childhood – depicted in the film of *Gone with the Wind*, in which a girl is shown with the sweat streaming down her face during an agonizing labour in which she later dies, and the French film, *Le Lit*, which showed a mother wincing with pain as the umbilical cord was cut!

degree of emotional security in childhood and the development of relations with her mother, father and siblings, the nature of the relationship with her husband, the image she has of herself as a woman, a wife and a mother, and the degree to which she can surrender herself to primitive instinctual pleasures and to the basic physical satisfactions associated with the health and well-being of the body and the harmonious functioning of her physiological processes.[1]

Childbirth with joy – entering into the process happily and deliberately accepting the task and adjusting oneself to fulfilling it – is as much a matter of the mind as of the body and is as great an emotional as it is a physiological process. Perhaps also it is as much a matter of unconscious as of conscious factors. Throughout this chapter we shall confront the *subjective experience* of the woman and the psychic factors to be taken into account no less than the physiological machine which she and her baby use together to bring the child to birth.

Moreover, in describing the feelings and behaviour of a woman giving birth to a child it is important to remember that labour is but one part of her whole psychosexual life. Puberty, ovulation, menstruation, love-play and intercourse, pregnancy, labour, the involution of the uterus in the weeks following birth, breast feeding and menopause – there is a flow and rhythm about her life bound up with her sexuality. The things she learns about herself, sensations of which she becomes aware, rhythms to which she is able to surrender herself, whether in reaching orgasm or in the remarkably similar urge to bear down in the second stage of labour, for instance, are interconnected. Where there is non-comprehension, or muscle spasm, or frigidity, then there tends to be a carry-over into other aspects of her psychosexual life, and I have known women who have discovered something about themselves in labour which has helped them towards a much happier sexual relation with their husbands afterwards. The emotional problems of childbearing are not separate and isolated, related only to having babies. They are an integral part of the fact of being a woman.

1. This ability on her part may be associated with her physical health.

This is where studies of uterine dysfunction of one kind or another sometimes prove very interesting.

Anything up to one fifth of women having their first babies have extra long labours. In all long labours there is a morale problem and it is important for husband and wife to be able to cope with the emotional problems that such a labour may present – the almost inevitable feelings of tiredness, the frequently encountered backache, which may be severe and may continue to a lesser degree between contractions, and the feeling of being utterly fed-up with the whole proceeding which may amount to a sense of angry frustration or despair.

Often there are good physiological reasons why labour has to be like that for those particular women; sometimes the baby is facing round the wrong way; frequently its head and body are not perfectly flexed into a neat little ball: sometimes the uterus does not do its work efficiently and for some reason fails to open the cervix adequately. Occasionally – but by no means always – the woman's feelings about her body and about childbirth seem to have something to do with this last problem of uterine inefficiency and *incoordinate uterine action*.

Studies of prolonged labours (over twenty-four hours) in which uterine action has been for one reason or another inefficient[1] have shown that these mothers tended to be of a certain personality type – that compared with mothers who had shorter labours and more effective uterine contractions they were inhibited, embarrassed by the processes that were taking place in their bodies, ladylike in the extreme, and endured what they were undergoing stoically as long as they were able,

1. See C. W. F. Burnett, 'Prolonged First Stage of Labour', *Nursing Mirror*, 29 July 1960. Dr Burnett found that the contractions often felt painful though they were inefficient in dilating the cervix. This was more frequent in first than in subsequent labours, with occipito-posterior presentations, and with large babies (over 9 lb.), and with hospital rather than with home deliveries. But often it occurred for no known reason. 'It has been found that patients who have prolonged labours tend to be reserved in manner, conventional in behaviour, with a desire always to be correct. When they have feelings of tension they characteristically repress them, in distinction to patients who have normal labours who betray any anxiety they may have quite openly.'

without expressing their anxieties. It was not these women's bodies that were causing them difficulties: they were being held up by the sort of people they were. They were not able to *give* birth.

A woman who is resisting and fighting her body can never feel delight in the tussle of labour. She lies in stoic patience and endurance, taut with anxiety, determined not to give in, even though there may be little or no real pain. She wants labour without sensation. For some reason which may have its origins in her own childhood, and which is probably linked with the quality of her marriage relationship, she is blocking her knowledge of herself and retreating from the overwhelming reality of the childbirth experience. Although pain may enter into the situation as the immediate and apparent cause of this retreat from experience, given a normal labour with understanding attendants and previous preparation for it, it would appear to be much more a question of personality adjustment.

It is asserted by some midwives that a woman shows her 'true nature' in childbirth and particularly as she reaches what may be a trying time at the end of the first stage. In the sense that a woman's basic capacity of acceptance or rejection of new challenges is demonstrated then, there is probably great truth in this.

There are some women who, long before they go into labour, state their intention of being deeply anaesthetized and not to 'feel anything'. They resolutely refuse to face up to it, even though they usually know nothing about the process except that it is supposed to hurt. Some others see it as an opportunity for exhibitionist suffering and enter it with a scarcely veiled delight, as did a woman who insisted that her husband should be present so that he could hear her screams and realize how she was suffering, and another woman who insisted upon the bedroom door remaining open so that her husband having his tea downstairs should not miss one syllable of her agony.

In a normal straightforward labour a woman's attitude of mind, her approach to the task that awaits her, and her preconceptions concerning the nature of the work that her body has to do, are more important than any sort of physical preparation she can make in advance. Whatever athletic exercises she may essay, however controlled her breathing, however complete her muscular relaxation, in the last resort the thing that matters most is, essentially, the kind of woman she is, and the sort of personality she has. That is why *preparation for labour cannot rest in purely physical training and in mechanical techniques of control and release alone*. Controlled muscular activity can assist her in making of her labour something she creates, rather than something she passively suffers, but her capacity for achieving this physical coordination is dependent upon her mind – upon her fearlessness and sense of security, her intelligence, her joy in the baby's coming, her courage, her self-confidence, and the understanding she has of herself. *The experience she has of childbirth is a function of her whole personality* and ideally the preparation for it carried on throughout the months of waiting should involve increased self-knowledge and a growing towards maturity.

One of the most useful pointers to the probability of a woman's success at having her baby with understanding and joy given adequate preparation and sympathetic attendants at the birth, lies in the marriage relationship, and the things which worry women most about their pregnancy and the baby's coming are closely connected with their husband's attitude to it all.

In this case, to those who have it shall be given. There seems a certain injustice in the fact that the happily married woman with her husband beside her at the birth is much more likely to enjoy her labour than the woman who feels that something is going wrong with her marriage. But, whilst it is not impossible for such a woman to have a joyful birth, the woman who feels she is alone in her pregnancy and that she faces motherhood alone, without her husband's participation or support, is at a grave disadvantage.

To a woman who is looking to her husband for help and loving understanding of her fears and hopes, a psychological withdrawal from the situation on his part is not only terribly disappointing, but may, if she was confident of his love for her, be a severe shock at a critical moment of their marriage. She cannot help comparing him with other husbands who welcome the birth of their child as an experience to be shared as far as possible with their wives. In such a case the woman must necessarily depend to a much greater extent upon the guidance received at the time of the birth from her midwife and doctor.[1]

But there is another type of husband who half-heartedly agrees to be with his wife at the birth if she really wants it but who is negative about the whole procedure, who refuses to read a book on the subject or to help his wife with exercises – who thinks, perhaps, that he is too 'manly' for this, or who finds it all too painfully embarrassing. Such a man may simply be ignorant of the sort of emotional upheaval that pregnancy and birth entail, and not have the imagination to understand his wife's need of him. Often the marriage is very young and the husband does not yet know his wife well.

The man who is not well-informed and has yet agreed to be at his wife's side is unlikely to know what he can do to help her and even a perfectly straightforward labour may be distressing for him. He does not understand what his wife is doing and feels completely out of place, and even though he is in the same room, the wife must feel a barrier of non-understanding. It is only fair to both that the husband too should have received prenatal instruction, and that he should be able to be of positive assistance, to anticipate her reactions, and to guide her in her task.[2]

To most women, I believe, the relation with the husband is all-important, and the relation with the obstetrician or midwife only secondary to this. But to some women, including some

1. Occasionally a husband who is very unwilling to be present will consent to be there if his wife insists. Each woman must judge for herself the wisdom of this course of action, but on the whole the very unwilling husband is best left out of the reckoning.

2. So closely is childbirth linked with the marriage relationship that, ideally, classes for preparation for expectant mothers should be much more closely associated with the work of the Marriage Guidance Council than with hospital out-patient clinics.

for whom the marriage relation is as yet unformed and immature, and with others of an older generation, the relation with the attendants becomes all important. This is particularly the case when a girl fixes her affection on a doctor as a father figure who must care for her and let her come to no harm – who will be firm, authoritarian and kind, like a loving father. One sometimes observes that during a woman's pregnancy she speaks so enthusiastically of her doctor and repeats his every phrase with such precision that it seems that the relationship is becoming an emotionally significant one for her. In her labour things will not go well until she has the security of his presence and feels his moral support, and it is important that he should stay with his patient if possible, as she depends upon him much more than the usual type of woman.

Other women need their mothers with them and turn back to them in girlhood dependence, and especially the daughters of a mother-dominated home do this, if they have not rebelled against it. The midwife may be a satisfactory mother substitute, especially if she is an older woman – and many women state their preference for older, more mature midwives, and worry in advance that a younger substitute will turn up when they are in labour. Even a sophisticated and intellectual girl may suddenly feel this need for an older woman on whom she can lean and whom she can trust absolutely. It is important, if the girl wants a mother figure during her labour, that she should have known the midwife long enough to have built up this relationship with her, and that the midwife should stay with her patient from the onset of difficult contractions, and not leave her, or introduce a substitute, unless another midwife is capable of filling the same role *vis-à-vis* the patient.

But, of course, not all women are like that. Many seek primarily a less highly charged relationship with the midwife – one in which the two can work as partners towards the safe and happy delivery of the baby. The mother comes to her task with specific training which complements the midwife's skills, and she looks to her not as a substitute mother in a situation in which she finds herself helpless, frightened and confused, but as the expert who can give her the right encouragement and guidance so that she can use to the full the tools she has for adjusting herself to the stresses of labour. Such a woman – and the great majority of those who have prepared themselves for childbirth by reading and by attending classes like this – embark upon a cooperative enterprise with a midwife whom they look to as a specialist to inform them, quite openly and truthfully, of progress and delay, and to remind them of what they should be doing at each phase of labour.

WHEN THE BABY IS DUE

Babies are sometimes born exactly 280 days after the first day of the last period, but many are born as much as a fortnight later and sometimes they are earlier. Only about five per cent of women have their babies on the day they were expected, and the majority have them about a week late. First babies are very often late.

Some mothers agitate for their labours to be induced if they think they are late, and some hospitals induce if the baby is as much as a week 'overdue'. This is particularly fashionable in the U.S.A. Medical induction may consist simply of the hopeful administration of castor oil, followed by an enema and a hot bath – which sometimes works – or (more likely nowadays in hospital) syntocinon or other synthetic hormone, in the form of an intravenous drip, or orally, sucked like a sweet. Syntocinon is a highly efficient way of inducing labour, and the doctor may decide to keep it going until after the delivery of the placenta. Sometimes syntocinon is used to restart a labour which seems to have come to a stop. One problem with this sort of induction can be that contractions are very intense, and sometimes each has two peaks, or each can have a sort of 'echo'. This can be extremely tiring for the mother. Surgical induction simply involves puncturing or rupturing of the membranes. Sometimes induction is required because of toxaemia or diabetes in the mother and for other equally serious reasons. (Then, of course, any discomfort is worth it in order to give the baby the best chance.)

The baby who is much overdue is at a disadvantage. The placenta gradually becomes less efficient in its functions and eventually, if the baby remains *in utero* sufficiently long, dies of old age. Some of the signs that a baby is post-mature are a very wrinkled skin, long finger-nails that need cutting immediately, and chalky white areas on the placenta. The baby born later than he should have been may need special care. But fortunately, these cases are few and far between.

It is important that the woman should get out and about in the weeks before labour commences, that she should maintain a lively interest in the world outside her home and that she should not sit indoors brooding about her state. When husbands and wives plan their recreations they should always include theatres, films, concerts and parties if possible for the weeks and days preceding the expected date of confinement, and the husband should have some sort of entertainment planned for the days immediately following this date, as the baby will probably not have been born by then and too many women feel depressed at this time. However, it is also important that the woman about to go into labour should have had sufficient sleep: so parties should not go on too late, and the mother should get a sedative from her doctor to enable her to drop off to sleep quickly if she is finding it difficult. (Boredom, worry, and over-tiredness are great threats to a woman's peace of mind as she starts the adventure of childbirth.)

Once labour starts, the body and mind seem to be flooded with energy and any weariness felt in the hours before disappears. Many women have started labour after a full day's work and yet have felt no tiredness. A warm bath,[1] relaxation, and some steady deep breathing will soon help to refresh the mother.

1. A scented bubble-bath induces a feeling of extravagant luxury, and if it is sufficiently bubbly prevents the mother from staring at her own abdomen watching for contractions.

LABOUR STARTS

Waves rise, each to its individual height in a seeming attitude of unrelenting competition, but only up to a certain point; and thus we know of the great repose of the sea to which they are all related, and to which they must all return in a rhythm which is marvellously beautiful.

In fact, these undulations and vibrations, these risings and fallings, are not due to the erratic contortions of disparate bodies, they are a rhythmic dance. Rhythm can never be borne of the haphazard struggle of combat. Its underlying principle must be unity, not opposition.

RABINDRANATH TAGORE, Sadhana,
The Realization of Life
Realization in Love

The signs that the preliminary labour period is beginning are well known: a 'show' of possibly blood-stained mucus (the gelatinous plug from the mouth of the uterus); odd contractions which feel something like menstrual pain: the painless rupture of the membranes, either slowly by leaking, or in a gush.[1] Any or all of these occurrences mean that the baby will probably be born within the next few days. Do not allow any of them to become signals for alarm. They are merely a sign that labour will begin shortly. Regular rhythmic contractions which dilate the cervix are the only true indication that labour is under way.

It is unwise to go to bed or to enter hospital until labour is well established, because then a woman tends to concentrate upon the inner mechanisms of her body before thinking about them can do any good at all. If she becomes impatient, it will help her to relax and is refreshing if she has a warm bath. She should go to the bedroom and get in touch with the midwife, who should have been previously warned, or ring up the hospital, as soon as she feels she wants someone with her other than her husband.

A woman can remain active and occupied – or, alternatively,

1. Frequently the membranes are ruptured artificially by the midwife. This does not hurt.

sleep – until she feels she needs to give her full attention to contractions. As contractions come, she should pause in whatever she is doing and follow the contractions with full chest breathing, rising to shallow chest breathing if she needs to. If she is standing, she should deliberately release all those muscles which are not necessary and feel herself hanging from the hips. If she has already practised relaxing while standing up this will come easily. Similarly, if she is sitting, she should release all those muscles she does not need to use and, leaning slightly forward with rounded shoulders, feel the lower part of her body as heavy whilst she brings her breathing into time with the contractions. She will find this simple also if she has rehearsed it during pregnancy.

The contractions come like waves, last between thirty and sixty seconds at first, and their crest is about two-thirds of the way through. The woman will probably find that the uncomfortable gripping sensation around her pelvis and any pain she may experience radiating in the lumbar area disappears completely once she starts doing the breathing she has learned and her husband is beside her rubbing her back, or very lightly massaging the lower abdomen. The regular rhythmic breathing will help her to control herself if she is very excited, whether or not there is any pain or discomfort.

It is important that she should start relaxing *before* she feels her body dominating her and before she finds it difficult to release her muscles during contractions. One should never try to talk during a contraction. As the first sensations of the contraction come she should *greet it with her breathing*. Take a full, deep breath, feeling the ribs swing out, without tightening the shoulders or chest, screwing up the eyes, or losing any of the active muscular release that one needs to maintain throughout labour. Let it go slowly. Rest on the slight pause that naturally follows. Take another – rest on it – and then let it go gently and easily.

With winter babies it is important not to get chilled during labour, as it is extremely difficult to relax when cold. The mother should wear a dressing gown and some wool socks or have a pair of warm slippers which she can easily slip on to go to the bathroom. Since she is likely to spend some time in the lavatory the heating should be left on there.

Women whose breasts feel heavy are usually more comfortable if they keep a well-fitting bra on throughout labour.

If labour starts when the woman is in bed she will probably be able to doze off and on for some time, but if she finds that contractions are sharp and wake her it is important that she wake herself up completely by splashing her face with cold water, drinking some hot coffee or tea, doing her face and hair, and getting things ready, or her drowsiness will make it difficult for her to control her breathing and relaxation.

These early contractions are sometimes more difficult than ones coming considerably later in the first stage, not because they have more force, but because the woman has not yet adjusted herself to receiving them. One mother who had been to my classes reported that she found it hard to control early first-stage contractions as it was very early morning and she was dozing between them, but when she woke up properly and started coping with her labour she found they were easy to deal with, and because of this, late first-stage contractions did not appear to be so powerful as these early ones.

If one bathes in the sea when the water is cold, putting the legs in first up to the thighs, they soon begin to adapt themselves to the icy water and to feel warm, but as one lowers the rest of the body into the water one realizes with a shock that it is icy cold. Whilst the legs had adapted themselves to the temperature of the water, the upper half had not yet had the time or opportunity to do so. It is the same with labour. A woman needs time to adapt herself to it.

The husband should check any signs of tension in his wife and should be the first to notice if she starts to grip the bed, to twist the sheet with her fingers, to screw up her face, curl her toes or stiffen her shoulders – or do any of the things which show that she is not completely at peace. Any contraction of muscles at this phase of labour is likely to be increased as labour advances and subsidiary tensions are built up in sympathy with the increasingly strongly contracting uterus. The mother cannot afford this dispersal of energy.

THE PRESENTATION OF THE BABY

The baby's skull is not hard bone all over. There are 'soft spots' or fontanelles – a diamond-shaped one at the front and another smaller one at the back of the head, with a narrow gap connecting the two. During the second stage of labour, the skull is moulded by overlapping of the bones at these cranial vault sutures. The larger one is called the *bregma* or anterior fontanelle, and forms a space between the frontal and parietal bones, and the smaller one at the back is called the posterior fontanelle, and lies between the occipital and parietal bones. Gradually, in the months after the birth, these ossify until the skull is all hard bone.

Obstetricians and midwives can, by internal examination, feel these fontanelles through the dilating cervix during the first stage of labour and in the birth canal during the second stage, and can so determine which way the baby's head is lying. The presenting part of the foetus is that part which can be felt through the cervix. Either the head, brow, face, or breech (buttocks) can present, the first being by far the most usual.

The more usual presentations

When labour begins the baby is commonly in an anterior or slightly lateral vertex position. That is, he is presenting by the head and the occiput is towards the mother's front, either lying on the left or the right side, the former position being slightly more usual. The obstetric terms for these are L.O.A. (left occipito-anterior) and R.O.A. (right occipito-anterior). The baby's head is usually well flexed forward on to his chest. His legs and arms are also flexed on to his body, and he is curled up like a hibernating dormouse.

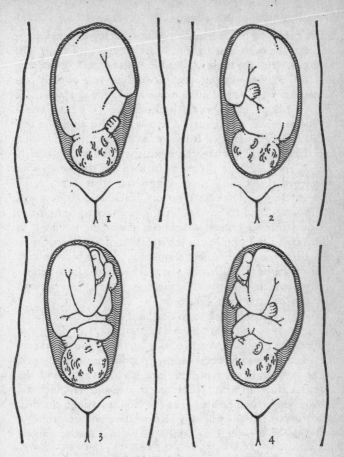

SOME POSITIONS THE BABY MAY BE IN
AS LABOUR BEGINS

Notice that these are all vertex presentations: i.e. the head is presenting.

1) Right occipito-anterior – R.O.A.

2) Left occipito-anterior – L.O.A. – the most common position. In both R.O.A. and L.O.A. positions the baby is facing the mother's back. These are very good positions for the baby to be in.

Some less usual presentations.

Some babies lie in a posterior position, facing either right or left, and the occiput is then towards the mother's back. The obstetric terms for these are R.O.P. (right occipito-posterior) and L.O.P. (left occipito-posterior). This is a slightly less favourable position and often means a rather longer and more tedious labour, more severe backache, and a greater strain on the maternal soft tissues. The mother with a baby in this position is best prepared for it by having it explained to her, and then she will not expect a rapid, easy labour. In the early part of the first stage she needs to keep her energy up with sweetened drinks and sugar lumps, or other light, easily digested foods. After three fingers dilatation it is best just to sip water, and to have nothing else either to drink or to eat, just in case general anaesthesia should be required, in which case a full stomach or the irritation of glucose could be very dangerous. In hospital, should the mother become very weary towards full dilatation she will be offered intra-venous glucose, which will quickly refresh and strengthen her and give her the extra 'pep' she needs.

The baby may be helped to flex itself further if she lies on the right side when the occiput is on the right, and vice versa, using pillows and the weight of one leg to support the uterus from beneath and to press on the baby to encourage flexion of the foetal spine. This position can also be assumed with the woman sitting up with the leg on the side against which the baby is lying raised on a stool or over the arm of the chair. In this position gravity will also help rotation and descent.[1]

A baby in a posterior position very often rotates into an

3) Right occipito-posterior – R.O.P.
4) Left occipito-posterior – L.O.P. – a rarer position. In both R.O.P. and L.O.P. positions the baby is facing the mother's front, and if the position persists (which it usually does not, since the baby rotates to an anterior position) he is born 'face to pubis'. These positions invariably mean a long first stage.

1. Vellay, who advises the use of this position, calls it 'the jack-knife position'.

anterior position at the very end of the first stage or during the second stage of labour, and mother and midwife have to wait patiently while this process takes place. If this occurs, it is the best possible thing that could happen. Rarely the baby begins to rotate but gets stuck in a transverse position (deep transverse arrest), and then help from the doctor or midwife is needed. When the baby remains in a posterior position this is known as P.O.P. (persistent occipito-posterior).

In face presentations (a fraction of one per cent of labours) the baby's head is not flexed on to his chest as it usually is, and unless the baby's head is small labour may be slower and some help may be needed with the delivery. In brow presentations the brow is presenting; this is very rare.

In breech births (about three per cent of labours) the first stage is often slow, although after the baby is born to the buttocks it is important that his head should slip out fairly quickly, so the doctor usually does an episiotomy to enable the head to be delivered more rapidly, though still gently and carefully.

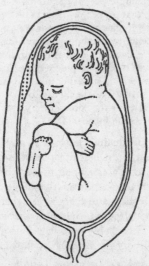

BREECH PRESENTATION

In breech deliveries a fully conscious and attentive mother can help her doctor a great deal by bearing down when she is instructed to do so.

However, it is not only a question of presentation. Most contractions flow like waves through the whole muscle of the uterus, beginning at the top and spreading downwards, getting stronger as they do so, and then fading away. Women do not usually feel the very beginning or end of the contractions, although they can be felt by a hand placed on the abdomen. Nor do they feel the sensations in the main body of the uterus – instead they get a concentration of feeling – a pull – over the cervix itself, and sometimes discomfort or pain in other places, such as the small of the back, or the thighs. It is not the contractions as such which may cause pain, but the stretching, thinning out and opening of the cervix which occurs at the height of strong contractions. In terms of function,

the normal uterine contractions have three important qualities. Not only does the wave spread downwards from the fundus, but the contraction of the upper part of the uterus is both more sustained and stronger than that of the lower part. This combination of downward spread, with longer and stronger contraction of the uterus, is called fundal dominance, and is essential for normal function. If the upper segment does not contract more slowly than the lower segment the cervix cannot be pulled open. In some cases of prolonged labour there is no fundal dominance, and the contractions of the lower segment are as strong as those of the upper segment. In other abnormal cases the contraction waves spread irregularly, and the contractions are incoordinate.[1]

If there is incoordinate uterine action of any kind the labouring woman may need a rest before labour can proceed normally, and if this is carefully explained to her she will understand that fairly heavy medication at this stage will allow her to sleep and be refreshed, and that she can then wake up and get on with her labour re-invigorated. If the incoordinate action continues she will probably need help with a Caesarian section or a forceps delivery, depending on how far the cervix has

1. *The Queen Charlotte's Textbook of Obstetrics,* 10th edn, Churchill, 1960.

managed to dilate. It is through no fault of hers that she needs this assistance; sometimes the machinery just does not work as it should. It does not mean that the same thing will happen with her next labour.

In primitive societies a woman with this difficulty might find a fire lit on her abdomen to smoke the baby out, or be beaten with sticks to force the child to emerge, or have to confess adultery, which is usually considered a barrier to spontaneous delivery. We have a good deal to be grateful for in modern Western obstetrics!

SEDATIVES AND ANALGESIA

Sedatives quieten a woman and help her to sleep. They are not pain-killers. Some midwives give them routinely to patients in the early part of the first stage, or those who start labour during the night. Anything but the mildest form of sedation is usually unwise with women who are using this method, since if contractions are strong enough to keep them awake they should be actively met and dealt with by controlled breathing and relaxation, and the woman asleep between contractions or in a very drowsy state cannot do this. As a result she may wake to severe pain which she never manages to eradicate, however hard she strives to adjust herself to later contractions. It is nevertheless important that she should not become exhausted from lack of sleep, and where for one reason or another labour is likely to be long, sleep, drug-induced if necessary, is essential. If labour starts in the night, with contractions further than five minutes apart, it may be a good idea to take whatever sedative has been prescribed to help the mother get to sleep in the last weeks of pregnancy, with a mug of hot milk with a spoonful or so of whisky, rum or brandy in it (the latter ingredient at least is for both parents) and to settle down to sleep again, with a hot water bottle, if liked, until contractions are sufficiently strong to need 'greeting' with the breathing. Even if one sleeps for half an hour or so, that extra rest is well worth while, and the couple have not spent the first phase of labour pacing the room, using up nervous energy, and wondering whether this is really 'it' or not.

A woman needs time to adapt herself to her labour, and to be led in gently by discovering that she can respond well to early and middle first-stage contractions. The absence of opportunity to adapt oneself gradually is a problem with some precipitate labours (those under five hours in total length). But in long labours it will not matter that a woman is losing sleep, if she is relaxed and using only the minimum of energy required to adapt herself to the contractions. One of the happiest labours I know lasted three whole days and nights; the woman did not require drugs since she was perfectly relaxed and completely confident, and her husband was with her all the time. But usually long labours are tiring.

One woman had a hospital confinement with a first baby and was given a sleeping pill when painless contractions were coming at seven-minute intervals at 3.30 a.m. – a normal and ordinarily praiseworthy procedure (her baby was not born till the following night at 11.30 pm.). She remarked afterwards, 'I wish I had not had the sleeping pill because they started to hurt then and I was too dopey to do anything about it. I kept on coming out of a doze and had more pain than at any other time.'

Whether or not sedatives are given early on, they should not be given late in labour unless it is prolonged and the woman needs sleep. If they are given then, she should have sufficient really to get to sleep, and she will wake refreshed and ready to get on with her labour.

Anaesthesia is of two kinds: general anaesthesia in which the patient sleeps, and regional anaesthesia which affects only part of the body. Regional anaesthesia is being used increasingly in obstetrics. Epidurals are one kind; they do not involve loss of consciousness, since only nerve endings in the area are deadened, and the woman just feels as if she were being filled up with iced water, and then perhaps a pulling sensation, from the waist down.

Analgesia is intended simply to deaden painful sensations. People react to analgesics in different ways, and an amount that makes one woman feel as if she has had slightly too much

to drink makes another pass out. On the whole, the more relaxed and fearless the patient the more effective is the analgesic
agent used. It must also be remembered by the woman who
has control over her breathing and is using her lungs to their
full capacity that she may inhale a much larger quantity of gas-
and-oxygen or trilene in a short time than a woman who is
breathing very shallowly.

Inhalation analgesia is available in this country for all
mothers requiring it. It can be taken by the mother herself,
who places the mask over her face and inhales through her
mouth. Often there is a hole over which she must keep her
thumb in order to get the effects of the gas, and as soon as she
becomes unconscious her hand slips away and she automatically takes no more. Women who have prepared themselves in
the Psychosexual Method can still use their controlled breathing when taking gas – and – oxygen, but will not be able to use
shallow chest or mouth-centred breathing when the mask is
actually over their face. To get the effects of both the analgesia and the light breathing, the best thing to do is to take
two good breaths of analgesia as the uterus comes into action,
and then, *putting the mask down*, to carry on up and over the
contraction with the breathing alone. Since it takes some
seconds for the effect of the gas – and – oxygen to be felt, the
woman thus gets the advantage of both. A small quantity of
gas-and-oxygen acts mainly as a relaxant and is useful for this
purpose. Taken in large amounts, it feels as if one is swimming
in treacle – or rather, dreaming of swimming in treacle. Some
people feel as if they are floating to the ceiling. Others just
feel a warm drowsiness stealing over them. [1]

Pethidine or pethilforan, with trilene and gas-and-air the
most commonly used obstetric analgesic agent in Britain,
is injected into the thigh. If given too early it tends to slow
down labour or even to stop it. Most primiparae (women
having their first babies) appear to benefit from a minimum
dose of pethidine or pethilforan[2] injected at about two-thirds

1. Gas-and-oxygen does not accumulate. Trilene, however, does.
2. 50 or 100 mgs., depending on the woman and the particular circumstances and her bodily state at the time.

dilatation, and (although it should never be injected as a blind routine measure) unless the mother feels that she is managing well without it, it is a good idea to accept it when the midwife suggests.

Pethidine or pethilforan is also useful when there is a tight rim of cervix which fails to retract, so that an anterior lip persists for a long time, and the midwife may suggest it then in order to help the cervix soften and draw up over the baby's head.

It is the custom in Britain to give trilene or gas-and-oxygen for as much of the first and second stages as the woman likes to have it. Whilst inhalation analgesia is obviously useful if a woman is suffering pain so severe that she simply must escape from it, and whilst it has certain beneficial psychological effects on the woman who is expecting it to help her, it has the disadvantage of imperilling a woman's control if she is endeavouring to have her baby by the method suggested in these pages. If she takes sufficient to make any significant difference, she is soon in a stupor, feels drunk, may talk at random, finds it impossible to synchronize her breathing with contractions, and cannot react directly to instructions from her attendants. Some women dislike this intensely, and have worse pain when taking gas-and-oxygen or trilene than when they are wide awake, controlling their breathing properly and having their backs rubbed.

For example, a woman having her first baby was given gas-and-oxygen when contractions were coming at two-and-a-half-minute intervals two hours before her baby's birth, and she said afterwards that she had felt she was losing control because 'I went to sleep as soon as a contraction was over' and she could not be ready to greet each new contraction with her breathing. Another woman, also having her first baby, wrote to me afterwards that during the transition phase between the first and second stage her midwives

kept suggesting that I should take gas-and-oxygen and eventually I said I'd try it. They kept telling me not to try to be brave and I couldn't seem to make them realize that I was not being brave and that it was bearable, with back rubbing. However, when I tried the gas-and-oxygen they could see that it didn't help me as much as back rubbing. In fact it made it much worse as I could feel everything but felt as if I was losing control. The backache was terrible and I couldn't stop pushing which I had been controlling by panting.

There are, however, many grateful women who say that they do not know how they would have managed without gas-and-oxygen. But it remains true, nevertheless, that *anything that tends to lower the threshold of discrimination of the labouring woman limits her ability to make full use of this method.* Ideally she should be given nothing that a car driver would not take before setting out on a night journey in fog, or an athlete before taking part in a race.

Only the woman herself can know if she really must have it, and it should be left to her to decide. It is the height of unconscious cruelty for a well-meaning but authoritarian nurse to press a mask over a labouring woman's face without giving her the chance to refuse it. On the other hand, a woman has not failed if she decides to take it. It has been her decision based upon her personal experience, and as such is the right one for her.

In conclusion, just as one would not attempt any skill one had acquired, such as driving a car, whilst semi-conscious or under the influence of powerful drugs, so in a straightforward labour a woman should not attempt the important business of having a baby in a doped state if she wants to use all her powers efficiently and to put into practice all she has learned during pregnancy. Marjorie Karmel in her book *Babies Without Tears*[1] describes how she was told in an American hospital when she was expecting her second baby that the effect of analgesia which she would be given would be simply that of having one Martini too many. She decided that she did not want to give birth to her child in that state.

Even if a woman chooses to have it at the end of the first stage it is most unlikely that she will need it during the second stage, although some women say that they went on taking it 'from habit'.

1. Secker and Warburg, 1959.

THE HUSBAND'S HELP

Throughout labour, the husband's watchfulness or that of whoever else is with the woman is as important as all the pre-natal preparations. Not only fear can lead to the tension which results in pain (Dick-Read's fear–tension–pain syndrome) – but also the worry that everything is not going according to plan, conflict with the attendants, or feeling that the atmosphere is unsympathetic. *Any feeling of frustration can interfere with relaxation and rhythmic breathing.* There should be no talking by any-one in the room during contractions. The husband should take over and deal with anything that needs arranging with the doctor or midwife, and with any explanations that may be required about the method of breathing the woman is adopt-ing or anything else she has learned in the classes for prepara-tion with which they may not be familiar. Usually midwives and obstetricians, even those who are basically unsympathetic towards this approach, will allow a woman to try things her way and say why they consider that another course of action is necessary, *if the husband is present*, and as long as he is not only knowledgeable about what his wife is trying to do, having read the same books and studied the same method, but is also tactful.

In hospital, if the husband has previously obtained permis-sion from the authorities to be with his wife and if she ex-pects him to be present, he should not desert her, and should leave her only when and if he is sure she can carry on happily without him.

THE OPENING UP OF THE CERVIX

The whole first stage is concerned with the opening up of the mouth of the uterus. The bands of longitudinal muscle fibre in the main part of the uterus are contracting whilst the cervix is gradually drawing up and apart, and its walls become thinner (see diagrams, pages 169-72). No voluntary effort can help this process. We have seen that midwives speak of the cervix as one, two, three, four or five fingers dilated – five fingers being full dilatation, when the cervix is completely opened, and becomes part of the uterus: uterus, cervix and vagina then form one canal. Some mothers are already one or two fingers dilated when they go into labour, the process of dilatation having started without their being aware of it. In most primiparae, as we have seen, the cervical canal has already been shortened and the walls drawn up during the three or four weeks before labour begins. In multiparae (women having their second and subsequent babies) the cervix is not usually taken up beforehand.

The dilatation is slowest during the first half of the process. That is, it usually takes a good deal longer to go from one to three fingers dilatation than it does to go from three fingers to full dilatation. Dilatation usually takes between eight to

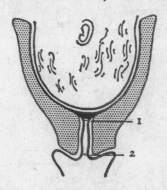

THE STATE OF THE CERVIX AT THIRTY-SIX WEEKS
IN A PRIMIPARA
1. Internal os.
2. External os.

The cervical canal is stopped up with a plug of mucus. During the last month of pregnancy in a woman having her first baby contractions of the upper uterine segment gradually draw up the tissues of the cervix and lower uterine segment. The cervical canal thus gets shorter and shorter until the cervix is of the same thickness as the uterine wall. The cervix is now said to be 'taken up' or 'ripe' for labour. In a multipara the cervix is often not taken up until labour begins.

twelve hours or more in primiparae, although they are not always aware of the beginning, and between six and ten hours in multiparae. But I have known primiparae who have had a first stage lasting twenty-four hours or more (in some cases without pain), and my first child was born in two and a half very pleasant hours, with some eight to ten painful contractions at the end of the first stage.

Once labour is really under way a woman wants someone, preferably her husband usually, with her all the time, and she should not be left alone. As each contraction comes it feels like a wave gathering in the distance. She automatically adjusts her breathing rhythm to meet it and as it comes towards her she 'swims' above it with careful, deliberate rhythmic strokes, right up to the crest; then she begins to feel it fade away and her breathing becomes softer, and she rests. At the end of each contraction she takes a few deep breaths in and out.

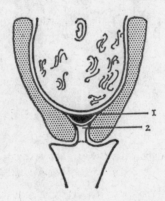

TAKING UP OF THE CERVIX
1. Internal os.
2. Membranes bulging.

The cervical canal may be seen to have been reduced in length.

Until contractions are coming at five-minute intervals or less, full chest breathing is usually sufficient to enable the mother to maintain conscious control over them and it is as well not to use lighter, shallower breathing until she really needs to do so. As she breathes in softly and slowly she feels her ribs spread out sideways, the whole bony cage expanding and the sternum lifted, and she continues this breathing steadily throughout each contraction. The woman herself does not feel the beginning of each contraction, although her husband may do so with a hand placed lightly on her abdomen, and can help her be ready for the next contraction by telling her when one is about to come. It is important that she begins her breathing before the height of the contraction is reached.

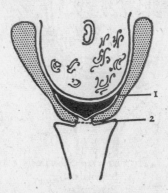

THE CERVIX COMPLETELY TAKEN UP

1. Internal os.
2. Membranes bulging.

This shows the state of the cervix early in labour. The canal has disappeared and some dilatation has already taken place.

When the midwife arrives she will probably prepare the woman by shaving the pubic hair, although in fact a woman can cut her hair short herself just before the expected date of confinement.

It is customary with many midwives to give an enema in order to avoid delay in labour due to the pressure of faecal matter in the lower bowel. A few women find this extremely unpleasant, and confuse the discomfort caused by the enema with labour pain. For this reason it is best not done unless it seems necessary to speed up labour (the enema actually stimulates uterine contractions in many cases) or unless the woman suffers from constipation, and then it should consist of plain water or saline solution only, since soap solution acts as an irritant. A few women are so worried that they will squeeze out faeces with bearing-down that it is better for them to have an enema too, as they are then less likely to do so. An enema should never be given towards the end of the first stage of labour since liquid faecal matter will then spurt out right

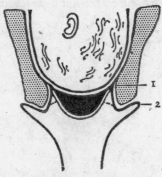

PARTIAL DILATATION OF THE CERVIX IN A PRIMIPARA

1. Internal os.
2. External os.

This cervix is about three fingers dilated. The intact bag of waters (the membranes) can be seen bulging through the cervix into the vagina.

through the second stage. A woman should relax when given an enema and use controlled breathing at the deepest level and slowest rate comfortable. She should indicate if she is having a contraction and ask the midwife to stop for a moment. There is no need to 'hold in' the enema. Nowadays a suppository is often used instead, which is much more pleasant.

It is important that the bladder should be emptied regularly throughout labour and the woman should remember to go to the lavatory, whether or not she feels she wants to, every hour. A distended bladder can cause acute discomfort as it presses against the cervix.

The midwife will tell the woman how far her cervix is dilated. This, as we have seen, is measured in fingers, although the midwife actually introduces only two. From three fingers dilatation, relaxation between contractions as well as during them is essential, and particularly release of the muscles of the abdomen and pelvic floor. When one is five fingers dilated the cervix is completely drawn up, and the second stage is about to begin.

The woman or her husband should ask the midwife about anything they do not understand at this, or any other, stage of labour.

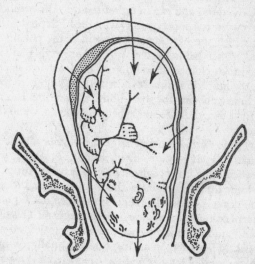

FULL DILATATION OF THE CERVIX

Full dilatation of the cervix is said to occur when it is sufficiently dilated to allow the presenting part, normally the head, but sometimes the buttocks (or breech), to pass through. The membranes have ruptured and the mother is now in the second stage. She is helping the contractions to press the baby down the birth canal.

Some midwives are disturbed at seeing women breathing more lightly and shallowly as labour advances and urge their patients to breathe slowly and deeply and to let the abdominal wall move.[1] The husband should explain to such a midwife that this is the method his wife has learned and carefully practised, and that to attempt to redirect her breathing at this late stage would only trouble her and threaten her self-control. The advantages of having previously discussed the methods of breathing with the midwife concerned are self-evident and any discussion of breathing methods should not be left until the woman is actually in labour if it can possibly be avoided.

The midwife is there as a counsellor and friend who can with an experienced eye watch for the different signs of the progress of labour and can interpret them to the parents and help the mother to cooperate fully with the birth process in the way for which she has prepared herself. If the parents have explained to her beforehand what they are trying to do by preparation for childbirth and do not confront her as an adversary, the midwife is almost invariably willing to cooperate with them in achieving the sort of birth they desire. Her name derives from the Anglo-Saxon 'a helping woman' – and that is what she is.

At any time during the first stage the mother may feel the membranes leak, or rupture and shoot out, sometimes with a pop; they feel like a warm, half-set jelly. Rarely they drop down and protrude from the vagina without bursting and look like a balloon heavy with liquid. There is between half a pint and two pints of colourless amniotic fluid inside them. This fluid is sterile, and automatically washes the birth canal from above downward. Whether they are ruptured naturally or by the midwife, the mother must *be prepared for an increase in the activity of the contractions immediately after*. They will become stronger and much more efficient and the intervals between them will probably get less. This is because the baby's head presses down more forcefully on the cervix. All the barriers have been eliminated.

1. One midwife objected that this method was 'too much like hard work'. But the point is that unless a woman is willing and emotionally capable of submitting passively to sensations which are acute and over-powering she must be prepared for hard work from three fingers dilatation onwards in order to meet the contractions and to cope with them.

The woman may find that in order to keep her breathing above the contractions she must now lift her breathing higher. She must be ready for this, and prepared to adapt her breathing to the new rhythm quickly. There may be a short period during which she does not adapt well, but she should not give way to despair. She must persevere to maintain careful control over her breathing and she will then find the right rhythm and type of breathing to meet these contractions.

Very occasionally labour begins and seems to be going well, and then suddenly stops. The mother, who has adjusted herself to the idea of being in labour and has made arrangements accordingly, is rather perturbed. After half an hour or an hour with nothing at all happening apart from some occasional twinges of backache and a heavy feeling in the pit of her stomach perhaps, she begins to wonder whether she is going to be stuck like this for days.

If this happens and the woman is not yet half dilated, she can get up and go for a walk. She should wear two sanitary pads just in case the membranes rupture while she is out, and, of course, should go with someone who can get her home or to hospital if labour suddenly starts to speed up.

When she comes in, or in any case if the weather is not suitable for a walk, she can have a warm, scented, luxurious bath and bask in it, but she should not lock the door.

Very often a pause of this kind comes before a sudden resumption of activity in the form of the waters bursting and the onset of late first-stage contractions.

SOME ACCOUNTS OF THE FIRST STAGE

Here are some women's own descriptions of what the first stage of labour felt like:

Second baby after a twelve-year gap:

Each contraction began with a glow of heat building up – as if an oven door was gradually opening – to a crescendo, then fading; one's rate of breathing seemed automatically to keep just on top of the wave of heat.

First baby, contractions every 4 minutes:

He made coffee and we heard the dawn chorus and watched the dawn come in – heavenly. We were completely at peace and loving every moment.

First baby:

With each contraction I held on to the arms of the chair and leaned forward slightly while my husband massaged my lower back and I did deep chest breathing and shallow chest breathing.... As each contraction became more powerful I smiled at my husband and this had a wonderfully encouraging effect and made me feel that I really could keep control.

First baby:

In the afternoon I did some washing and in the evening we went to the theatre. On the way home a little bit of water broke, but so little that I did not think it could be 'it'. So we went to bed. At about 11.45 I had the first contraction. Soon others followed. They started at five-minute intervals and were quite strong. I did not want to spend too much time in the hospital before the baby's birth and thought for a first baby I certainly had many hours to go. But when the intervals became still shorter my husband rang up the hospital and we went there about 1.30 a.m. The Sister examined me and said I was already fully dilated. I don't know when I did that!

First baby, 9 lb. 4 oz.:

The midwife arrived to find me almost 3 fingers dilated. The midwife and her pupil stayed with us but gave us perfect peace to work quietly together. I was using shallower breathing and still found great relief and even enjoyment from having the lower abdomen massaged gently.

First baby, posterior presentation (contractions coming every 5 minutes or less):

A cushion in the small of my back almost completely removed backache. (It was noticeable how ineffective it was to try breathing without proper relaxation which I was doing before, and getting myself worked up as a result of thinking I couldn't cope!) The waters started to leak so we called the midwife. She shaved me, examined me, gave me an enema. Funnily enough I found all this soothing rather than otherwise. I vomited which also made me feel better.

Second baby, posterior presentation 2–3 fingers dilated:

I continued to potter around all day, without the contractions becoming strong enough to require much in the way of positive relaxation. So long as I kept on the move they kept coming at 2–7 minute intervals, but as soon as I sat or lay down they became much milder and slowed down to 12–15 minutes, so I had to keep going for little walks, doing gentle spring-cleaning etc.... I rang the midwife, saying that we didn't seem to be getting anywhere, as contractions were not getting any stronger. Midwife arrived and decided that on the contrary I was fully dilated.

First baby:

Dr C. ruptured the membranes. What a marvellous feeling! Gushing, warm and refreshing. Contractions were becoming strong and powerful. I found the most effective way to handle them was to take one or two deep breaths and immediately switch to the shallow rapid breathing. For the latter half I found gradual breathing down, upper-middle-lower lobe, more effective. Sometimes I found blowing out very helpful even though I wasn't yet in transition. I visualized one of three mental pictures: the diagrammatic pattern of breathing for a contraction-wave; the uterine muscles effacing and dilating the cervix; me sitting on the crest of a wave coming into shore at a beach on the Isle of Crete.

Second baby, after a traumatic first labour:

Contractions were coming about every 2 minutes, one strong and the next one not so strong. Whilst putting baby clothes to air and water to boil, I found the best position was to bend over anything of suitable height with feet apart.
(This was a 2-hour labour.)

Second baby, of a doctor's wife, after a traumatic first labour:

I enlisted my husband's help and although I felt he still secretly thought I expected too much of childbirth, he encouraged me and when the time came was a marvellous help. At about 4 I asked my husband to phone the midwife, as I was sure I was getting on quite

quickly. The contractions were very fierce and about every 3 minutes, lasting 1–2 minutes, but with him there to steady me I breathed my way over the top of them, and I had difficulty in persuading him I was getting on jolly fast! Once or twice I lost the rhythm and then they really did hurt badly.
(Baby delivered just before 4.30.)

First baby, posterior presentation:

I spent the rest of the first stage on my knees and elbows with my head resting on my arms during contractions. They were coming quite strongly every 2 minutes and I was using shallow chest breathing and occasionally pelvic rocking. The doctor found me 4 fingers dilated.

First baby:

The contractions gradually moved up to 5-minute intervals and the backache increased although the contraction as such was not painful. We decided to go to hospital. The contractions rapidly moved to 1–2 minute intervals and my husband was a great help by counting the seconds in my ear so I knew just when the height would come.

First baby:

The contractions were down to every 3 minutes and lasting about 1 minute. Now they were getting a bit uncomfortable – but not unbearable. This is where I found the breathing helped tremendously. Also my husband and the nurse took it in turns to rub my back.

First baby:

The pain in my back lasted only about 30–40 seconds, seemed to reach a peak about half way through. Bill rubbed it, and together we did shallow rapid breathing.

Second baby after traumatic first labour. This one proved to be a posterior presentation and 9 lb. 6 oz.:

Contractions were now coming every 2–3 minutes and I was making the most of all three stages of breathing and relaxing. I did find blowing out helped a lot to keep the rhythm of shallow rapid breathing going smoothly.

First baby, posterior presentation. A husband reports:

I found J. looking relaxed and happy. Contractions came at slightly varying intervals, but generally every 4 or 5 minutes. I spent most of my time massaging her back and giving her her barley sugar stick to suck. I had to leave to lecture and as J. had not yet been examined, the nurse arranged to do so before I left. They were very surprised to find her 3 fingers dilated. Her breathing was still fairly 'low down'. She rode most of the contractions well and rhythmically, except when one caught her unawares. She found massage of the back and the insides of the thighs most helpful. While I was away a student midwife took over the massage. I returned to find the position much the same. But the baby had rotated itself.

First baby, posterior presentation which rotated spontaneously:

I was having contractions at 4-minute intervals. My backache was uncomfortable, and C. massaged it and the inside of my thighs, which helped a great deal. I felt perfectly able to cope. I also had a hot water bottle in the small of my back, which helped. I was advised to lie on my left side, as this would help the baby to rotate. The nurses kept on asking me whether I wanted pethidine, and if not why not.

First baby, 3-hour labour:

I was so aware of the baby's head pressing on the rectum and I think it was probably the most uncomfortable sensation of all. I found the position on all fours with pelvic rocking in between contractions very comfortable. When I arrived at the hospital I tried to time it so that I had a contraction in the car – and then get upstairs before the next one came. The lift wasn't available for some minutes. I sat on the stairs – had a contraction and the membranes ruptured.
(The baby was delivered half an hour later.)

Second baby, 8 lb. 9½ oz. (first also born with preparation):

My mother-in-law said she'd make a cup of tea for me, so I came down to get it and had another contraction half way upstairs as my husband came in. He rang the hospital as I was having the next contraction, and the waters broke with a ping and a splash on to the bedroom floor, and I could feel the baby's head pressing *right* down, my body wide open, and there was the second stage. I called to L. and told him there wasn't time to get to the hospital. I'd have the baby in the bathroom, it was so difficult to walk! (I was so silly.) All I wanted to do was wash my briefs, as the mucous plug and show had come away and I didn't want to leave them for in-laws to find; the other thing was for poor L. to scrub the carpet where the waters had shot out. We did all this before the next contraction. (Labour lasted one hour.)

Other, and fuller, descriptions of labour by husbands and wives form the central theme of my *Giving Birth: Parents' Emotions in Childbirth* (Gollancz, 1971), and readers may like to refer to this and get a more cohesive picture of the experience of labour as it exists for different women.

CHAPTER 9

The Climax of Labour

Is it beyond thee to be glad with gladness of this rhythm?
To be tossed and lost and broken in the whirl of this fearful joy?
RABINDRANATH TAGORE, *Gitanjali*, lxx

THE END OF THE FIRST STAGE

THE contractions are at their most fast and furious between two-thirds dilatation and the end of the first stage. The sensations are strong, overpowering, and can be at the same time delightful. One is swept away like a little boat at sea in a great storm of exultant emotions and a tremendous sweep of physical energy. The body takes over in what seems a wholly marvellous way. It kneads and squeezes; contraction follows contraction powerfully and with precision. Indeed, in spite of the strength and the relentless force of its action there is a delicate accuracy about its workings at this time. One can only be in awe and deliver oneself over, in faith, to this wonderful thing – one's own body at the work of creation.

It is extremely difficult to describe adequately what a woman in labour feels at this time. I have tried to describe my personal sensations. Most women would probably say that the sensations were painful for at any rate part of this time, but mothers I have prepared for childbirth usually remark: 'but not impossibly uncomfortable', or 'quite bearable', or say that they could 'keep on top of the contractions' with their breathing. Women interpret these sensations in such different ways that whereas one mother will say calmly, 'I did have pain, but it was nothing to speak of, and I felt quite happy', another will seeks words to express these sensations by saying, 'It wasn't at all painful. It felt as if I had a warm fire inside me. I could feel a glow as each contraction came', and still another will feel so glad that at last she is in labour that she will remark, 'It hurt, but it didn't matter.'

As a woman approaches two-thirds dilatation she may find that she starts to shiver uncontrollably, and she may vomit. The shivering can be lessened, at any rate, by warm coverings, hot water bottles, perhaps an electric heating pad (covered with a waterproof fabric), socks or stockings on the feet and massage of the adductors. (See page 109.) A woman is especially liable to vomit if she has eaten once dilatation has really started. She can often avoid sickness by taking only sips of liquid once labour is under way.

Except in fog or very cold weather, or when a premature baby is expected, it is as well to leave the windows open until delivery is imminent, as the fresh air is good. The mother should adjust her position until she is comfortable, and may find that she wants to be in different positions at different phases of her labour. During the late first stage she will probably need help in doing this as she may feel very heavy and almost fixed to the bed. She may well find that the front lateral which she has practised during her pregnancy is especially comfortable, or may prefer to be on her back with the knees bent. These are the positions perhaps most commonly adopted, but in both cases she should be well supported with pillows so that she can really relax in comfort.

The contractions get stronger and stronger and appear to have a reckless intensity, the intervals between them growing shorter, until they are down to two minutes or less. They bring with them acute abdominal tension and one feels rather as if an enormous balloon was being blown up inside and then slowly deflated.

At this point the mother may choose to receive a minimum dose of pethidine, but often she feels that she needs no pain-relieving drugs at all.

She has probably lifted her breathing higher and is doing quick breathing at the height of each contraction now. It comes to her much more easily than when she was practising it during her pregnancy. If she has not yet altered her breathing rhythm so that it is lighter and higher the husband may suggest to her that she does so, and can help her by breathing with her. At the end of each contraction she breathes deeply and rests completely, and uses the interval between contractions to check that she is really relaxed.

The midwife may want to examine the mother vaginally or *per rectum* every now and then to see how far the opening of the uterus is dilated. The cervix hangs like the clapper of a bell inside the birth canal, so she can feel it with her fingers. She should let the mother know the progress she is making. It is not sufficient to make what one mother complained of as merely 'soothing noises'. This examination need not hurt at all, especially if the mother remembers to relax and after taking a deep breath breathes out whilst the midwife inserts her gloved fingers, and at the same time releases the muscles of the pelvic floor.

It is better not to be examined during a contraction, as one wants to concentrate on it and one is too preoccupied towards the end of the first stage with shallow rapid breathing. If the midwife attempts examination *per vaginam* during a contraction one should ask her to wait a moment, or the husband should be alert to request this. If the mother keeps her eyes open she can easily indicate by shaking her head or lifting her hand that she would prefer the midwife to wait a minute.

The midwife may suggest to the mother that she should listen to the foetal heart-beats with a stethoscope – a very encouraging and thrilling sound to hear at this time.

The patient can be examined in the left lateral or Simms position, which entails, if she is already lying in the front lateral with her face to the left, simply drawing up her left leg towards her breast and rounding her back, with her buttocks either at the end of a divan bed or at the side of a bed which has headboards. She can then easily revert to her previous position without having to move her weight once the examination is completed.

Obstetricians and midwives sometimes prefer to have women in a dorsal or modified lithotomy position for examination. In this case the woman lies on her back with her legs apart and knees bent. Usually in hospitals this position is preferred. In the true lithotomy position the woman's legs are raised in stirrups. This is, of course, only possible in hospital.

If her attendants prefer her to lie like this, and this is often favoured during the second stage, and if she is comfortable, it is easier to remain in this position, as it is a nuisance to have continually to readjust one's position. However, some women find that they suffer from painful cramp in the legs in the true lithotomy position. In this case they should tell the nurse and lower the legs on to the delivery table, raising them when the doctor wants to examine.

Some mothers like to lie on their backs, their head and shoulders slightly raised with pillows, with the lower part of the spine flat, and legs flopped apart and well flexed during late first-stage contractions. This is an excellent position for this phase of labour. Others experience pain in the thighs at this point, which can be relieved by either gentle or very firm massage up and down the upper legs from the pelvis and back to it again. Either the woman herself or her husband can do this. She will have to lie on her back in order to be massaged in this way. Occasionally pain is centred around the pubis and groin, at the very base of the abdomen. Very light massage, using the fleshy pads of the fingers with a circular rhythmic movement, by the woman herself, will help to relieve this. Here again she will have to lie on her back.

It is important that however drowsy the woman may feel *between* contractions after three fingers dilatation – and this drowsiness is nature's way of achieving muscular release – she should be fully awake at the onset of each contraction and stimulated to cope with it actively by deliberate stripping of tension from her body and by regulating her breathing to harmonize with the wave of contraction.

Sometimes a woman feels disconcertingly cut off from reality, and hates the feeling. It is rather as if one were in a space-ship and had lost contact with earth, with none of the usual points of reference, in a timeless, limitless existence. It is exacerbated by loneliness, isolation and the monotony of continually recurring contractions in a long-drawn-out labour. Some women happily accept this sensation of drift, but others fight against it.

A condition known as *kayak-angst* has been described among

Eskimos. When the Eskimo hunter is out alone on a calm sea paddling or sitting quietly, there develops a lowering in the level of consciousness brought on by the absence of external reference points at a time when the hunter is engaged in simple repetitive movements or sitting motionless, and staring at the sea. He gets confused and dizzy – and even the psychologists who were studying this found that they were disturbed in exactly the same way when they tried to do it, too.

This condition may arouse vivid memories in some women who have been alone in a hospital labour ward for any length of time, lying with nothing to see but the ceiling and a tiled wall, sometimes with a light shining in their faces.

The situation in labour is, of course, rather different, because the effect of stimulatory deprivation (through loneliness, silence, postural immobility, confinement in a small room, bare surroundings, often unpatterned and clinically white walls) is coupled with intense stimulation from one organ of the body, the contracting uterus. In such cases the result can be a failure of nerve.

It is important to create points of reference, therefore, in case this sort of stress should occur and threaten a woman's equilibrium. The labouring woman should not be left alone unless she wishes it, and should be able to see a clock, or watch, and wear glasses if she requires them. Familiar objects, the presence of her husband or a midwife or doctor she already knows and likes, the use of phrases she is familiar with to help her remember what she has learned and to keep relaxed control, and reference to the preparation she has received, so that she is reminded that she has rehearsed it all before, are important. When she feels shivery, or says that she does not want her baby today, or wants to go home now, or that she just wants to sleep and forget her labour, she should have someone there to remind her that these are all normal occurrences in a labour that is going well, and are, in fact, signs of progress.

TRANSITION BETWEEN THE FIRST AND
SECOND STAGES

Gradually the woman feels the nature of the contractions change. They may become irregular, and she gets a catch in her throat at their height. She realizes that the expulsive reflex is beginning to establish itself, though she is probably not yet fully dilated and should not push voluntarily. In fact, only when the desire to bear down is *completely irresistible* must she permit herself to start pressing the baby down the birth canal. It may take quite a long time – half an hour or more – and in some women it never establishes itself in its full force. In any case, whether or not the woman deliberately decides to push the baby out by her own exertions, it will get born.

The woman is still doing shallow rapid breathing and may be in considerable discomfort which makes her irritable. Since at this phase of labour her conscious mind cannot really decide what her body wants to do unless she is very well prepared and capable of great control she feels a certain conflict in the situation, wh ich may express itself in annoyance with her attendants or her husband, and occasionally a wish to 'get away from it all', to escape her labour and the inevitability of the process. She protests. 'Oh, do go away and leave me alone' or 'I only want to sleep'. No woman need feel she has 'failed' if she says something unkind to her husband at this point, but on the other hand the fact that she knows she may possibly behave like this involuntarily should not predispose her to permit herself irrational behaviour at the height of labour.

A slight and perfectly natural developing amnesia is often further reinforced by drugs of an analgesic nature and especially by inhaled gas-and-oxygen or trilene, and under these conditions it is usually much more difficult for a woman to control the impulse towards flight by conscious redirection of her thoughts in a more positive channel, by decision to enter into her labour rather than to try to avoid it. This is one of the reasons why analgesia creates its own difficulties and does not in itself form a solution to the problem of pain in labour.

If she seems to be escaping into a dream world – which may be more one of nightmare than of pleasant fantasy – it is important that her husband should seek to bring her back to reality by stimulation. He can wring out flannels or sponges in very cold, preferably iced, water and rest them against her forehead, cheeks, lips and the nape of her neck with each contraction. As the woman is probably feeling rather sticky and hot by now this is refreshing anyway and is usually greatly welcomed. He can help her loosen the bedclothes and adjust her position until she is more comfortable.

Some women, especially those whose babies are in an occipito-posterior position, have severe backache during this phase and whilst massage often relieves it[1] the mother may find that it is more comfortable to be on all fours, with the legs and arms apart, taking the weight of the baby off the spine, and resting it on the front of the pelvis, and some women like to rock the pelvis slightly forward and back during a contraction. A few women prefer to kneel with legs wide apart and sitting on their heels, leaning forward to rest with their head on pillows between contractions. Others prefer to retain their front lateral position. Often a hot water bottle, or a polythene bag filled with ice, relieves backache.

If the husband is unable to rub his wife's back, she can herself press the knuckles of one hand against the sacro-lumbar region where the pain is. Some women benefit greatly from firm regular massaging of the adductors. This is of particular help if the woman encounters difficulty in relaxing her legs, as some do when they get 'shivery' at any time from three fingers dilatation on. If legs jerk at all during contractions, or if she curls up her toes, it is certain that her legs are not completely relaxed. She should have extra light-weight blankets on her, bed-socks, and a hot water bottle, bottles at her feet and also *between the tops of her legs*, and massaging of the legs during contractions.

Very rarely the cord prolapses, and then it is important to relieve pressure on it by allowing the baby's head or whichever part is presenting to fall well away from the bony rim

1. Dick-Read described this as 'the pain period of labour'.

of the pelvis between contractions. The midwife may suggest to the mother that she kneels, leaning forward with her knees near her chest, if this rare contingency occurs.

A shift in position may in itself be sufficient to remind a woman of her purpose. But the husband can also tell his wife that before very long she will be holding the baby in her arms, that this is considered one of the most difficult (if not the most difficult) phases of labour, but that it rarely lasts more than about half an hour and soon she will be able to engage in her labour more actively.

Some women start gasping as the contraction reaches its height. In this case they should quickly blow out and start breathing rhythmically again, and should be firmly reminded to do this. It helps if the husband sits beside his wife and breathes with her to give her moral support and to remind her of the need for respiratory control and muscular release, and to keep her eyes open and on him during contractions. A woman who has been doing shallow rapid breathing with her lips apart for some time always requires a sip of water to moisten her dry lips and mouth. However, she should not drink so much that her bladder becomes distended as this can slow up labour by creating a sort of traffic jam inside her.

Occasionally the urge to push comes very suddenly and more or less overwhelmingly, and the woman has not time to adjust to it; this may occur even when the woman's cervix is not completely dilated to allow the passage of the baby down the birth canal. Then she needs extra control over herself. This is achieved by blowing out hard at the height of the contraction: that is, when the urge to press down becomes almost irresistible. Thus a rhythm is established – and it may have to last for a dozen contractions or more – of shallow breathing mounting to the crest of a contraction, when the woman blows out quickly for as many times as she needs to when the urge to push reasserts itself (possibly three or four times during a contraction), and then continues the light, rapid breathing until the contraction fades away.

Frequently the rim of the cervix fails to retract equally all round the advancing head, and a part of it – at the front – is caught up over the baby's head for a few minutes or occasionally longer. This is known as 'an anterior lip'. It is particularly common with posterior presentations. The mother wants to bear down but must not yet do so or she risks injury to the cervix. Continued forceful pushing against an incompletely dilated cervix can make it puffy and swollen so that the opening, instead of getting wider for the baby's head to come through, is actually made smaller, and labour is held up. The best thing to do is to stop pushing and wait patiently for full dilatation. This is when previous practice in blowing out when the urge to push is at its most compelling proves to have been well worth while. When a woman is adequately prepared this probably helps her more than gas-and-oxygen at this difficult phase of labour. The untrained woman is usually given gas-and-oxygen to stop her pushing.

The woman will hear her own breathing becoming rather noisy, but should not let this distress her nor feel the need to apologize to her attendants. This slightly noisier breathing is perfectly natural and *is not an indication that she is in pain*. If she keeps her chin well forward on her chest, and keeps her breathing *as light as possible*, she will sound less desperate. If at any time the bearing down urge becomes too strong to be dealt with in this way, *it is all right to push*.

SOME ACCOUNTS OF THE TRANSITION PHASE

This is how some mothers coped with this phase of labour:

First baby, posterior presentation:

The midwife said there was just a crescent of cervix to dilate. I asked if this was an anterior lip and she said 'Yes'. I found this very cheering because although the breathing was coping very well with contractions, the backache was bad. I must say that apart from the backache, thanks to the breathing, I never felt anything that could be called painful.

Second baby, posterior presentation:

Things began to get a bit hazy, and I got the 'far-away' feeling from then until the actual birth. I found it a tremendous effort to say anything to anyone, even when resting in between contractions.

First baby, 9 lb. 4 oz:

I found relaxing a little more difficult here but I was wide awake and fully in control. For ten minutes I delayed bearing down by using shallow rapid breathing punctuated by crisp blowing out. My midwife thought this was quite splendid. No thought of pethidene or gas-and-air entered my head.

Second baby, first also with preparation, 8 lb. 9½ oz.:

We swerved up to the hospital at 5 to 4. I couldn't help wondering whether I was imagining it, as these were very very mild contractions too with no sudden point of almost uncontrollable pushing. They were like first-stage contractions in shape, and the breathing was like this: puff, puff, puff, blow, blow, blow, *blow, blow* – BLOW – very slow and steady blowing out. And that would be the end of the contraction. They hustled me into a chair and trundled it along the corridor to the delivery room. The labour was still fantastically mild. I asked if I could push – or rather, explained why I was blowing out, and Sister said, 'Oh any time you like, just push'. I said I didn't want to push against an insufficiently dilated cervix. She came across and said had my husband been to classes and nodded to the other midwife to bring him in. She said, 'Your baby's just sitting here, waiting to be born.'
(Baby born half an hour after arrival at the hospital.)

First baby:

I didn't want him to massage me or even to talk as I needed all my concentration, but it made all the difference in the world having him there. Then the contractions started to change – a kind of surging feeling rather than a real urge to push.

First baby, posterior presentation:

I began to have a desire to bear down at the height of them. I did the pant – pant-pant-blow – pant-pant-pant-BLOW rhythm and they were manageable.... My husband had my hand and as they began I gently moved it and we did them together so I could keep the rhythm up. They were difficult but it was exciting as we felt we were coping.

First baby:

The urge to bear down was terribly strong – I had no idea it would be as strong as that – and without C. there keeping me 'under control' I would have lost my breathing completely. He reminded me to blow out when I felt the urge to push, to breathe rhythmically, and to be patient – a thing I found difficult! I did not find it easy to relax my legs, and they felt a bit cold in spite of my long white socks.

THE SECOND STAGE

The second stage is that of the expulsion of the baby. The vagina lies almost at right-angles to the uterus, and by the onset of the second stage uterus and vagina have become one open birth canal. Women often enjoy it, and the pleasure it brings is similar to the simple delight in defecation that one can witness in a small child, and is a reminder of once vigorous infantile pleasures which have often been repressed in the adult and have become taboo – which may in itself threaten the inhibited woman's composure. When the bearing down reflex is fully established the urge to push is compelling and irresistible. Some women are horrified at the intensity of the desire to bear down. 'It is,' as one mother commented afterwards, 'a very primitive sort of urge. I was astonished that it was so strong.' Women who have been inadequately prepared for the passion they feel welling up in them in labour may try to escape from the sensations. They panic and grip themselves in pain, resisting the urge with all their might.

But the second stage need not be at all painful. It is often pleasurable even for unprepared women who can enjoy co-ordinated muscular effort. If the woman is capable of this and is not pushed beyond her powers by over-enthusiastic attendants who take on the role of cheer-leaders rather than patiently and quietly standing by, there is no reason for it to be anything but exhilarating and very satisfying for the woman who knows what to expect and how to use her body. Gas-and-oxygen, although it is sometimes taken by women who felt they needed it for the transition phase between the first and second stages and who continue to take it, as they admit afterwards, 'from habit', or because they are 'scared', and not because they are in pain, is unnecessary and undesirable for the healthy woman who has been previously prepared for labour.

In the second stage the baby, who has often entered the pelvis some weeks before labour starts, passes right down through the pelvic arc; this descent and expulsion being not in a straight line, but a gentle curve, since the uterus is almost at right-angles to the vagina. It helps if the mother visualizes this arc when she is bearing down.

The position for the second stage which the mother is likely to find allows her the best play of muscle in pressing the baby down the birth canal is on her back, propped up by three or four pillows at an angle at which she can observe the crowning and birth of the head comfortably, with the base of the spine flat on the bed, in the relaxed posture of Titian's Danaë. Since pillows may slip as the mother bears down, it is best for the husband to sit on the left of his wife, and to put his arm behind her head or just below her shoulders so that she can press back against it as she pushes. He can then sit close beside her, encouraging and talking quietly with her between contractions, and they can watch the birth of their baby together. It is a much better place for the husband to be here than segregated in a far corner where he cannot kiss her or hold her hand, which is the custom in some hospitals where the husband is allowed to be present at the delivery, and it has the added advantage that the husband does not get in the midwife's way.

Many domiciliary midwives are accustomed to have the mother lie on her left side in the Simm's position, but even if they prefer this for the actual delivery they are often very willing to permit the mother to go through most of the second stage in the dorsal position (on her back, propped up). Sometimes if they have a firm mattress on which to deliver they have no objection to the mother remaining in this position.[1]

If the woman cannot get the correct technique of bearing down, she will amost invariably be able to do so if she squats and pushes in that position for a few contractions. In many primitive societies women have their babies in this position. The pelvis is at its widest when the mother is squatting.

It has been generally accepted until quite recently that this was a time of enormous effort and muscular straining for the mother, and the classic picture of a woman in the second stage of labour was that of the mother grunting and groaning with effort, the sweat streaming off her face, veins standing out on her forehead, lips pressed together, eyes glazed and the skin red and hot, whilst her attendants stood by and exhorted her to still further efforts. Women were told that they must work hard, that this was an athletic achievement which demanded strength and persistence, and that they would feel tired out after the delivery. In fact, even in otherwise easy labours, mothers who had struggled to use every ounce of energy did feel exhausted after the delivery; their lips were parched, their eyes bloodshot; they felt weak and only wanted to be left alone to sleep. This is still the situation in many hospitals and home confinements today, and it has become routine to expect the mother to want to go to sleep after her labour – which nearly always surprises trained mothers who feel fresh and very wide awake.

So intimately was the idea of physical exertion associated with childbirth that still in the first quarter of the twentieth century some midwives and relatives used to urge the mother to push, to 'lean on the pains', long before she desired to, and before her cervix was effaced, thus putting extreme stress upon the transverse cervical ligaments, which often became torn, and sometimes producing an oedematous cervix through which the baby's head could not pass with ease. This resulted in a

1. It is worth discussing the position for the second stage and that for delivery with the midwife or obstetrician early in pregnancy so that the mother may practise in the position she will be in in labour.

delayed second stage or in a high or mid-forceps delivery. Roller towels were tied to the bed-posts for her to pull on and the whole process became a formidable display of strenuous effort. Since then it has come to be generally realized that the mother must not be permitted to push until her body is ready for it, until the baby's head can be seen and the way is clear for its expulsion, but even now some midwives and obstetricians want to get the baby born as soon as possible once the second stage has really started, even when there are no signs of foetal distress, and exhort the mother to push yet harder. If the mother shows no signs of wanting to push, she is often told, 'Just try a little one, dear, and see what happens.'

The idea of birth as an athletic achievement – the simile drawn is that of rowing – is still current in France, where it has been revived under psychoprophylaxis. Under this system the obstetrician may keep up a running commentary on the progress of a woman's labour, and although some women like this constant encouragement, some are distressed by the continual flow of words, the reiterated, '*Alors! Madame, attention! Poussez! Poussez. . . . Poussez. . . . Poussez. . . . Encore! Encore! Continuez! Continuez! . . . Très bien. Très bien. Reposez-vous. Respirez bien*' etc.[1] It is very doubtful whether the management of the second stage has yet reached its ideal form in this system.[2]

The better the coordination of uterine contractions, voluntary muscular activity and breathing rhythm, the less effort is required from the woman and a relaxed and natural second stage results. The important thing to remember is that one should *listen* to contractions in order to remain sensitive and aware of their exact nature, and be alert to any change in their character. The urge to push varies greatly from contraction to contraction. One pushes exactly when and as long and as strongly as each indicates. It is a little like the orchestra responding to the conductor's baton. The contracting uterus is the conductor.

1. Lamaze has made a record of a labour conducted by himself. It is interesting to compare this with the record of a birth by Dick-Read.

2. The films of labour conducted by Vellay are much more peaceful than Lamaze's record.

The researches of Constance Benyon[1] indicate that babies get born satisfactorily and with less need for forceps deliveries and for episiotomies when the mother economizes in muscular effort and when she is permitted to follow her own inclinations, when 'pushing' is not mentioned by her attendants and she is not hurried at all. Constance Benyon started her investigations after noting that cardiac cases, who were not allowed to strain in labour, had their babies just as easily as normal healthy patients, and she discovered that the more perfect the coordination the less conscious effort was needed and the less expulsive force was required, because the resistance presented by the pelvic floor was minimal. Only irresistible pushing was necessary, and only the minimum of that.

The woman who has learned bearing-down assisted by contraction of the diaphragm must remember that however conscious, voluntary and controlled her actions when she was practising, when it comes to labour this sort of action will come quite naturally. The point of learning how to do it beforehand is that delicate coordination between the muscular actions and the contractions is necessary in labour, and she is more likely to have full confidence in herself and to trust her own body if she knows what is happening and does not rely upon commands coming from other people, but can interpret her physical sensations and know how to react to them instantaneously, without doubt or hesitation. Moreover, the woman who has learned beforehand the nature of the muscular activity she is called upon to perform in the second stage of labour does not tense up muscles that are not involved in the process of expulsion. She learns how to keep her shoulders rounded forwards, her chin tucked in against her chest (she often forgets and her husband should tilt it foward for her), her jaw relaxed, her arms and hands loose and, above all, the muscles of the pelvic floor released as she presses the lower part of her spine flat against the bed as she pushes, rounding rather than arching her back, and so automatically rocking

1. Constance L. Beynon, 'The Normal Second Stage of Labour', *Journal of Obstetrics and Gynaecology of the British Empire*, vol. LXIV, No. 6, December 1957.

the pelvis forward. After each contraction she relaxes completely.

The woman who has not received previous instruction, or in whom it has been inadequate, is liable to push her chin in the air and strain her neck and shoulder muscles, clenching her fists, and sometimes also arching her back and tensing the muscles of the birth outlet. As she strains down she groans, such is the tension around her throat. She is not only wasting valuable energy, but she is actually presenting an obstacle to the baby's birth in that she is tightening the pelvic floor and putting great stress upon the connective tissue which supports the walls of the vagina.

Frequently, if a woman who is getting weary and desperate, and is pushing ineffectively, simply stops *trying* to bear down, and allows herself to ride the contractions with mouth-centred breathing, the urge to expel the baby establishes itself in force, and she cannot help bearing down after a short time. She comes to realize what her body demands of her, and tackles the remaining contractions with fresh energy and enthusiasm.

When a woman knows what she is doing she steadies herself for each contraction by taking one or two deep breaths as it begins. There is a slight pause in which she observes the character of the contraction and the sensations it gives her. As it rises towards its height she will know whether or not she must push with that one, and whether she must push, but only gently. If it is a powerful one she will find that her breath is held involuntarily and that her ribs and diaphragm become fixed, just as she has rehearsed it in class, and that she pushes down on the uterus with the diaphragm, and relaxes the abdominal muscles. This pressure comes entirely from above and she does not tighten at all below.

SOME ACCOUNTS OF THE SECOND STAGE

First baby:

This stage ... was not painful at all even when the head crowned. My husband sat at the head of the bed with his arms round my waist to support me. I was very comfortable. I was not in the least tired.

There was no pain at all. I could feel the baby's head behind the rectum like a very hard lump. Between contractions I was so completely relaxed that I could not answer when anyone spoke to me. I know I was using the contractions well and the midwives remarked on this and how well I relaxed.

First baby:

I began really to enjoy the birth. It was a wonderful thing to be able to use the power of the contractions to make the baby come. I suppose I have never worked with such a sense of power and assurance of success.... A most satisfying and rewarding experience.

First baby:

It was the most wonderful work, but very hard. My husband soon could see the head. [The nurses felt she should take gas-and-oxygen and placed the mask on her face] but I kept pushing it away, saying, 'No thank you; I have no pain. I have no use for that.' I don't think I would have enjoyed the birth so much with it.

Second baby, after a very painful first labour:

The second stage was easy. Two magnificent pushes – no wasted effort there.

First baby:

I can honestly say I felt no actual pain, though I had slight backache.

First baby, at onset of second stage:

Oh, isn't this exciting?

Third baby:

I thought I could feel the wedge of waters pushing its way down the birth canal, and simultaneously the strong urge to push. The midwife ruptured the waters whereupon the head pressed on the perineum and she asked me to pant. The rapid shallow breathing came easily. The next push produced the baby's head.

First baby (a trial labour in which everything was in readiness for Caesarian section if necessary. The mother, however, delivered the baby spontaneously):

It was marvellous, it was such a beautiful rhythm. G. [her husband] said 'Breathe in, breathe out, breathe in, fix the ribs and diaphragm, and push,' with each contraction, and sloshed cold water on my face in between contractions. He had his arm behind my head and held it forward for each contraction. I had oxygen and that was a great help. I got in four pushes for each contraction.

First baby:

What an exhilarating feeling to be able to push at last! With one contraction either I didn't take in enough oxygen, or I pushed harder than the contraction demanded of me and felt very dizzy. Water between contractions to moisten my mouth and lips, and on my face, refreshed me tremendously – very invigorating. There were five or six contractions. They varied in length and rest interval between them. The strength of the contractions varied too; some demanded terrific pushing effort; for others moderate effort sufficed. For some contractions I pushed three or four times, others just once or twice.

A father's comment:

I could see the top of the baby's head coming down. It looked like a sump of oil.

Second baby:

I just adored having her. I can't wait to have another baby (my husband says I'll be producing them until the menopause!). I found the expulsion much more easy this time as I knew just how to push. I wasn't a bit tired at the end, only very happy and relaxed.

First baby:

Everything came so natural and perfect that I easily surprised myself.

Second baby:

It was pain, yes, but without the fear and tension that normally accompanies physical pain. I think my husband felt that too. He said that it was a wonderful experience. We were together in something very real and fundamental. I expect the nurses thought I was quite mad because I kept telling P. that I loved him, and wanting him to kiss me, in between pushes . . .

First baby, after a very prolonged labour, with the baby changing position. Taking gas-and-oxygen:

Although I could still feel everything it made me feel very relaxed and happy and was a great boost to my morale. . . . I was roused by a simply huge contraction and I became much more alert. Very soon after this I suddenly started pushing, quite involuntarily, right at the end of a contraction. From then on things went simply splendidly. I felt the pushes were very effective but there was no undue strain and no pain. At first I got a little muddled with my breathing but soon established a rhythm and then got two or three good pushes in with each contraction.

First baby, posterior presentation:

I suddenly became very wide awake and the next forty-five minutes were full of hard work and excitement. Two young medical students arrived. I suddenly realized that the midwife was explaining what was happening in great detail for their benefit as she never would have bothered for me. The time just flew by as it seemed I made enormous progress with each push.

First baby:

The second stage started with a bit of a 'cheering act' but then I was allowed to push when I felt like it which was infinitely better.

First baby:

The feeling of the head on the floor of the perineum is strange; it was like a ball coming through an opening not quite large enough, and falling back each time to try again and this time to get a bit further. It wasn't painful: certainly it was uncomfortable, but no more than that. It could also be likened to a wave washing up on the sea-shore, coming a bit further each time.

First baby, 9 lb. 4 oz.:

The time came for bearing down. I must say that I found this was quite hard work and found it rather nice to be able to push back against my husband. We had the wedge and had suitably arranged the wardrobe mirror and set up a lamp which allowed me to see every centimetre of the birth outlet very clearly.

We thought the head was appearing but Dr L. explained that it was really due to the membranes still being intact and baby's floating hair visible behind them. The bearing-down movements were strangely pleasurable although I do remember saying rather anxiously to the doctor, 'I do hope I shan't tear,' but he was very reassuring. My husband helped enormously to see that I breathed rhythmically at this very exciting stage. [She had no laceration.]

Another husband's comment:

I could see the baby's head coming, wet and wrinkled – like a winkle.

Second baby, posterior presentation, spontaneous delivery:

The midwives had asked me from time to time whether I felt like pushing, but had not urged me when I said no. When the urge *did* come, I was surprised by the strength of both the involuntary muscular movements and the voluntary effort that one put into it. The uterus certainly did 'set the pace', and it seemed quite natural to fit in my efforts with what the uterus was doing at the time. I had rather severe backache during each contraction, but it did help tremendously to be able to be doing something positive towards the birth.

Second baby:

Once in the second stage I was away. I enjoyed every moment of the half-hour and found the bearing down not nearly such an effort as I had anticipated, and *far* more enjoyable than climbing a mountain. Each contraction seemed to dictate the amount of effort required and I just left my body to do the work – no mental energy was needed. My husband held up a mirror for me to see the first appearance of the baby's head.

Second-stage contractions, then, are normally but not invariably greeted with deep breathing. Mouth-centred breathing is used, however, if the midwife wants the mother to 'blow the contraction away', punctuated with the crisp blowing out of the transition phase breathing. In this way the too rapid descent and delivery of a baby's head can be slowed up. (Babies can be born too quickly, not only too slowly.) Mouth-centred breathing is used in all cases of precipitate labour, or simply of precipitate second stage. Some babies practically fall out, and there is an art, both for the mother and for the midwife, in delivering them gently and slowly. This should be done by control of the urge to bear down rather than by holding back the baby's head, which is always bad.

Grand multiparae, women who have already borne three or four babies, especially if they are fairly close together and are not very old yet, *may* find that they have this sort of labour. (On the other hand they may be fatigued with too much housework, broken nights and the constant pressures of the family – and the uterus itself can be tired and slack – and have a long-drawn-out labour. One can never bank on any special sort of labour in advance.) Their pelvic floors may also be much softened, and this means, not only that the baby will pass through them easily, but that the muscles themselves should be given gentle treatment. It is therefore wise for them to approach the second stage of labour prepared to do mouth-centred rather than deep breathing, with deep breathing simply at the end of the contractions.

It must be emphasized that the precipitate second stage, if it is quick because the mother is expelling the child too forcibly, can be bad for both mother and child. If it just happens that way, because the mother is relaxed and *lets* the baby be born, this is a very different matter.

Sometimes the perineum is seen to become rigid and shiny as the baby's head distends the pelvic floor. In these circumstances it is more than ever imperative to slow up the process so that the pelvic floor has time to dilate gradually and can take the passage of the baby's head without a resulting laceration or the necessity of an episiotomy, unless for the baby's sake it is essential that he should be born quickly, which happens in some cases. Occasionally uterine contractions in themselves are so strong that little can be done about it, but the mother should push *only when the urge to push is irresistible.* She should endeavour to stop pushing entirely and *should*

*pant lightly for the next few contractions and blow out as they reach
their peak*, in order to control the desire to bear down until
the perineum is no longer taut. In this way the birth outlet
will probably dilate so as to permit the birth of the baby's
head without a tear.

As the coccyx and sacrum are pushed up and backward by
the pressure of the baby's head passing over the pelvic floor the
woman may experience temporary backache and try to adjust
her position in order to get more comfortable, in vain. She
should welcome it, since it means that the baby is already much
lower. In cases of posterior positions of the baby's head the
backache is likely to be much more severe. She may feel the
bump which is the baby's head move down with each contraction and recede again slightly at its termination. This is uncomfortable to the extent that it feels like a lump in the mattress
or a knot of blankets which have got tangled underneath
one's back, but is not painful.

The mother feels the pressure of the baby's head against the
rectum as it proceeds still lower and reaches the deepest point
in the arc of its journey. It feels very much like a grapefruit –
and indeed has something of this consistency, since the bones
of the baby's skull slightly overlap each other at the fontanelles
in order to ease his passage into the world. The moulding of
the baby's head noted immediately after birth results from
the pressure of the birth canal, and the nature and extent of
the stresses put upon it by the uterine contractions and by the
mother's efforts during the second stage.

If the woman is pushing hard because she feels this is what
is *expected* of her in the second stage and not because her uterine conditions demand it, or because she senses an atmosphere of haste or urgency, or if she is pushing against an as yet
inadequately dilated perineum, the feeling she experiences will
be one of extreme discomfort. This, of course, cannot always
be avoided in the case of women with tough and resistant
perineal muscles and particularly with women over thirty who
are having their first baby, or in the case of an exceptionally
large baby.

Although these few moments tend to be quickly forgotten

after the birth of the baby they are not pleasant and many women feel it was the time when their self-control was most threatened. They felt they were 'going to pop' and described the sensation as 'preposterous'. In a second stage which is progressing gently and rhythmically, however, there is no sensation which one would wish to forget afterwards.

As soon as the baby's head crowns the mother must be ready to stop pushing, even though she feels like it. Then the head will be born more gently. She may be able to feel or, if she is watching, can see herself when this happens and will stop. If she is not yet aware that the birth is imminent – too busy bearing down – or if for any reason she does not want to look, she must be prepared to stop immediately the obstetrician or midwife tells her to. She can then look down and see the first glimpse of her baby. Seeing the baby about to emerge into the world will make her so happy that it will not be difficult for her to relax then.

THE DELIVERY

The morning stars sang together, and all the sons of God shouted for joy.

The Book of Job

The crowning is commonly believed to be one of the most painful moments of labour, and many unprepared women approach it with dread. Some babies' heads do not crown. If the mother is pushing down hard and without sensitivity, ignoring the dictates of her uterus, and if she fails to wait for the gradual dilatation of the perineum, the head may pop out like a cork out of a champagne bottle instead. The mother's perineum will then be torn and repair will be necessary. With the ideal delivery however, the crowning of the head, its birth and subsequent birth of the body all take place slowly and gently.

The woman begins to feel herself gradually opening up, like a bud into full flower, a strange experience which may be rather frightening for an unprepared woman. This may be accompanied by a warm tingling sensation as the baby's head begins to make the perineum bulge forward. The feeling is very acute and some women hate it; they find it what can only be described as 'shocking'. It is a sensation so vivid that they do not know whether it is pleasure or pain, whether to welcome or retreat from it. For some it is almost as if they are being violated, and here there would appear to be some link between sexual adjustment and the woman's ability to accept her physical experiences and to welcome the activity of her body in labour, and particularly so at this moment preceding delivery. The woman who is adequately prepared – both physically and *emotionally* – for the experience of labour, greets these sensations which herald the baby's birth with delight.

Since the head is the largest part of the baby the vulva is then stretched to its widest capacity, and often remains so for several minutes till one, two or three contractions have pushed the whole body out. If the vulva is not dilating naturally the person who is delivering the mother may do a quick episiotomy during a contraction, and then the baby's head can slip out easily without injuring the mother, leaving a small straight cut rather than a jagged tear, which can without difficulty be sutured later. There is no reason why an episiotomy should mar the joy of childbirth and mothers need not be apprehensive about it nor let its possible performance introduce anxiety into the labour. Although ideally it should not be necessary, undoubtedly under the circumstances of modern life it is often desirable for the sake of the future health of the mother's pelvic floor. With this method of preparation, however, everything possible will have been done by the mother herself to permit the birth outlet to dilate naturally and easily, and I know of mothers who have borne first babies exceeding nine and ten pounds in weight who have suffered no injury to the perineum.

The obstetrician may inject to anaesthetize the outlet and a few still put the mother out as the baby emerges, but not often in this country. He often gives a local anaesthetic, similar to that given by a dentist for drilling a tooth, before he does an episiotomy, although most mothers who need episiotomies are numb already because of the pressure from the baby's head.

For the conscious woman who is participating actively in labour, the moment when the head crowns is an intensely pleasurable and very exciting one.[1] There may be a high degree of desensitization of the perineum because of the pressure of the head, and the sensation, though acute, is not one of pain but of extreme pressure. If the baby's head is large and the pressure great, the mother frequently feels nothing except a 'bulge', since the perineum is numbed completely by the great pressure. With smaller babies and rather more room, the mother often feels more, and is able to observe sensitively each separate part of her baby as it uncurls from the birth canal. The crowning comes much sooner than one expects, either with a contraction or the mother may be asked to bear down *between* contractions, and when she sees the rounded shape of her baby's head and its damp, dark hair she suddenly forgets about herself entirely and is concerned only for the child. The baby's head looks amazingly large and if she knew nothing about the mechanisms involved she would probably wonder how it was going to get out. It continues to rotate so that it presents the narrowest diameter and can slide out easily. This part of the birth must not be hastened and she must use conscious control to be patient and allow the baby to be born by uterine contractions without any forcing on her part. Immediately the head has crowned the mother can ask the midwife, 'What do you want me to do with the next contraction?' If and when the midwife wants her to push or to squeeze gently she will certainly tell her. Otherwise she should take it for granted that she should *not* be bearing down.

The mother should pant lightly and 'breathe the baby out',

1. Like many other teachers of prepared childbirth I used to tell mothers that they would feel 'a splitting, burning sensation', until one newly delivered mother wrote to tell me that she had not felt anything like this and that it had been pleasant. After that I described the sensations of bulging without adding any suggestion that the crowning itself was not to be enjoyed, and since then have discovered that few mothers have complained about it. In fact in nearly every case there is no reason why it cannot be a thrilling and very happy part of delivery.

but if she is actually watching the birth she is probably so interested that she will not need to do this for longer than a few seconds, and I notice that many mothers I have prepared find themselves talking to the baby or to their husbands at this time. The mother who is lying completely flat on her back or is insufficiently curved forward in the left lateral and hence only partly aware of the actual birth, may find it very difficult to control herself at this time. In order not to push she should concentrate on doing the panting breathing she has learned, and if even then she feels an almost uncontrollable urge to bear down during contractions she must blow out hard whenever the sensation becomes very strong. She will find that she *can* control herself and allow the birth to be gentle and unforced.

But the mother who is sitting up or is propped up at an angle of between 40° and 60°, or even one who is lying on her left side and is curved well forward to watch (although this is more difficult) may *see* exactly how far she can give, and if the outlet is not artificially anaesthetized she can *feel* the point at which the baby's head must be eased out more gently. This is so even more if the midwife is not massaging or guarding the perineum, which is the custom of some (but which the mother can ask her to stop if it is bothering her). This is also a very important few minutes for the midwife, who wants to get the delivery perfect. It is understandable if sometimes a young and not very experienced midwife gets excited or a note of panic creeps into her voice, and the parents should not allow this to worry them. The midwife rarely needs to touch the child's head, given a gentle, controlled delivery of this kind.

All this time it is very important to relax the muscles of the birth outlet. They should feel soft and suspended like a hammock. And the mother should actively release them so that she feels as if she is helping her baby's head to bulge through. Remember that the function of the birth canal is precisely this – for a baby to be born through. This is what this part of the body was made for, and the equipment a woman has is very efficient, so she should relax and let it work.

The woman feels as if her whole body is becoming a gateway into the world for her child. The head begins to ooze out. She may be asked to squeeze gently *between* contractions to help this process. The gates swing back and open wide. This is the moment of triumph and exaltation. The baby is sliding down. The head is born to below the chin. It looks very blue, even purple. The child has not yet taken its first great gasp of air into its lungs. If, as sometimes happens, the cord is twisted around the neck, the midwife will unhook it with her finger, or clamp and cut it immediately. First the anterior shoulder is born, and then the other comes out. The baby's warm damp arms rest on the mother's thighs and then the whole body slips out, wriggling and soft. But even before the body is born the chest may flutter and then swell and the child may open wide its mouth and cry – a high-pitched wailing scream. He suddenly turns red, and the mother gasps with pleasure at this, his first greeting, his first reaction to being thrust into life and out from the warm, swaying comfort of her body. She wants to take him into her arms immediately to hold him tight and soothe him. The child's legs slither out and his screams get louder and louder, and all the muscles of his little body seem to be clenched in protest, in indignation at being born. His mother laughs; he looks so annoyed, so helpless, his rage is so futile, and she wants to protect him from himself and his own violent emotions. Whether boy or girl she realizes that this child is exactly what she desired.

The midwife waits for the cord to stop pulsating so that the child may get all the blood possible. The fingers of her left hand rest on the cord, her right hand grasping the scissors with which she will cut this gelatinous mass, which is twisted round and round like a barber's pole or a malacca cane and sometimes even loosely knotted, giving evidence of the activity that the mother felt inside the uterus, and the way in which the baby kicked, bumped, squirmed, twisted, somersaulted, and swam in her body like a fish in the sea. The cord is tied or clipped in two places and cut about four inches away from the baby between the two ligatures. Sometimes the midwife allows the husband to do this. The child is now a separate individual.

THE BABY'S APPEARANCE

The baby may be covered with a white creamy substance which has been protecting his delicate skin *in utero*. This *vernix* gradually washes off, although it is rarely completely removed at the first bath. Some midwives think this affords a valuable protection in the first few days of life and do not attempt to remove it. Sometimes babies have fine hairs all over their skin, the *lanugo* which also appears to have afforded protection *in utero*. One notices it over the baby's arms and in the small of his back and low over his forehead and at the sides of his cheeks. This hair gradually falls out. The first crop of hair on the head usually also disappears to be replaced by a new crop which may be of a different, and often lighter, colour. As this happens some babies look as if they are getting red haired.

Occasionally the membranes have not ruptured over the baby's head and the child is born with a caul like a cap over the vault of the skull or even over the whole head.

The baby who has not been doped by the mother's anaesthesia or excessive analgesia usually cries immediately. It is important that a child should breathe as soon as possible after birth, as otherwise there may be damage to brain cells due to lack of oxygen. Between 35% and 67% (according to different research studies done) of babies of doped mothers do not breathe immediately at birth, whereas only 2% of babies of mothers who have received no anaesthesia or analgesia do not breathe immediately.[1] The midwife and obstetrician have various techniques which enable them to get the baby to cry, and so to breathe. Usually all that needs to be done is to clear the mucus from the airways, and it may be sufficient to hold the baby upside down so that it drains out. The midwife wipes the baby's eyes, nose and mouth with swabs; he is bundled in a warm towel or blanket and is handed to the mother, who holds him in her arms, marvelling at the perfection of every detail, the tiny shell-pink finger-nails and the faint eyelashes and brows. The child clutches her finger firmly in his tight grasp and may go to sleep on her breast.

1. H. B. Atlee, *The Gist of Obstetrics,* Thomos, Illinois, 1957.

THE THIRD STAGE

Meanwhile the placenta has usually detached itself from the lining of the uterus and has slipped down into the vagina, waiting to be expelled by a gentle squeeze, or there may be further uterine contractions to expel it. Rarely the uterus needs help to expel the placenta and then the midwife may press on the mother's abdomen. Occasionally the placenta follows the baby right down, and merges with him in one big bundle.

The placenta, red and meaty, is criss-crossed with blood vessels. The midwife examines it and puts it in a bucket. It can be burned in a dustbin or boiler, or buried in the garden. The uterus quickly contracts, and hour by hour sinks lower in the mother's body till in ten days or less it is no longer an abdominal but a pelvic organ. After six weeks it is back to its normal state, or, in the case of a first baby, is a little larger than it was previous to conception.

After the baby is born the mother will have some discharge. This *lochia* is evidence that the lining of the uterus is repairing itself. For the first day or so it is usually bright red, then it turns pale pink for a few more days (or sometimes weeks) and finally she may only notice it after she has breast-fed the baby. The stimulation of the breasts results in contractions of the uterus (which she may feel as 'after-pains', which can be uncomfortable and for which she may need analgesics and a hot water bottle over the lower abdomen). These contractions associated with breast-feeding are important in restoring the uterus rapidly almost to its former size, and, hence, in the mother's speedy and complete physical rehabilitation. Early ambulation encourages rapid drainage of this lochia from the uterus.

Most mothers, in my experience, find it very difficult to use a bed-pan in the hours following delivery and are more comfortable if they get out of bed and squat over a light-weight bucket. After that they are usually able to go to the bathroom if it is on the same floor. It is normal not to want to empty the bowels for four or five days.

SOME ACCOUNTS OF DELIVERY

First baby:

I felt the baby slide out gently. There was no sensation of splitting –
just a gentle opening up. The baby cried. I asked to hold her hand.

First baby:

I saw the head when I sat up for the next contraction. That was
marvellous. Then the mouth opened very, very wide and he yelled.

First baby:

It was wonderful. I had three contractions for which I bore down.
John [her husband] helped in delivering her, and she was born
screaming.

First baby:

The head appeared and I looked down to see it and then another
contraction and it was well through. Still no pain or even a feeling
of stretching – it just felt rather hard. . . . The baby was born and
there was still no pain and it was very thrilling to see it being born
and hear my husband say it was a girl. She yelled loudly as soon as
she was born, and the cord was cut and I held her.

First baby:

I could feel her kicking and heard her first cry. It was the most
wonderful moment in our lives.

First baby – on seeing her baby's head ooze out and rotate:

Oh how adorable! Oh darling, how adorable! It's my baby!

Third baby:

Panting made me feel really secure at the crowning. I looked down
as the head was being born and heard him cry while his body was
still inside me. It was very exciting – for my husband too. He really
enjoyed it. . . . The baby was laid on my abdomen feeling warm,
wet and full of life.

First baby – the husband comments on his daughter's birth:

I shall never forget the look on her face as the baby slipped out. It was wonderful. Triumph, well-being and joy.... One could never capture it in a photograph.... It was the most wonderful experience. It is the sort of thing I shall never forget.

First baby, high forceps delivery with caudal anaesthesia:

The doctor nicked the rim of my cervix and the baby was delivered by forceps. My husband saw her born, and particularly enjoyed watching her uncurling as she came out of the birth canal. He told me her sex. I was very excited and felt nothing of the birth except a sensation of pulling during the delivery.

A father's comment:

All I could see was a tiny portion of the baby's head lightly covered with black hair. My wife and I took a breath and bore down. 'Bear down honey; it's coming, bear down, bear down, hold on, hold on.'
    Then the glorious moment when the little being was wholly released from the vagina. 'It's a girl,' I shouted. 'It's a girl, honey!' I was beside myself with joy. I had given birth along with my wife. It was glorious, just glorious. We are so very happy. This experience has made a bond between us that no ordinary birth, nor in fact any experience, could have done. Turbulent and passionate as it is – we are so blessed.

The mother of a second baby, after a traumatic first labour, as her baby's head crowned:

Oh ... it's *nice*!

First baby, breech:

Then suddenly there seemed to be lots of people and activity and the stirrups and everything were brought in and I felt suddenly very awake.... I was told then I was to have an anaesthetic as there was some risk involved for the baby and so of course I left it entirely to the doctors.... I really got going. I know I managed to have a good bit of the bottom half of him myself. Then they gave me the anaesthetic. When I came round again I could hear the baby crying and could hardly believe my ears. My husband came in and in fact saw the baby first, which was lovely.

First baby, posterior rotated to anterior at end of first stage. The husband:

I was standing behind the bed and found this a wonderful moment. She had had no analgesics throughout and looked relaxed and wonderfully happy: all her mind concentrated on this little creature, and her arms reaching out lovingly for it. This is a time for husbands to value and treasure, of tenderness and fulfilment.

First baby, 9 lb. 4 oz.:

The head crowned. The midwife told me to pant at once and I did so instantly. A few more very gentle pushes produced baby's head (my husband was breathless with delight and excitement) and soon her whole body wriggled out and M. cried out, 'It's a little girl,' and clasped us both rather ecstatically, during which time the placenta emerged with a few further pushes. Catherine cried at once but it was necessary to remove a little mucus. The pupil midwife did the delivery and she was highly excited but I felt she handled it so very delicately. This was her first domiciliary delivery. Dr L., Miss P. and Nurse W. had enjoyed the delivery and were all amazed that we had produced this large baby without tearing.

First baby, posterior till onset of 5-minute second stage:

The vulva stretched. It was a very nice feeling, very pleasurable. It stretched well. I stroked his head when it crowned. The head came out; I didn't tear; I saw it become bigger and bigger. It was a beautiful feeling of warmth. I got so excited. My tiredness disappeared. It was lovely.

First baby, deep transverse arrest. Baby 10 lb. 2 oz. Forceps delivery with local anaesthetic for episiotomy:

I was not at all anxious, and J. was behind me giving me encouragement. The doctor offered me trilene which I refused. I was very relaxed and still smiling and talking as he inserted the forceps. It was a wonderful sensation as I knew that within minutes baby would be out. The birth outlet felt warm and soft and the only feeling I had of the forceps was like when you rub your fingernail along a comb, not at all unpleasant. With the next contraction I pushed and the baby's head was born, the size of a pumpkin, not a grapefruit, as it had a caput. I put my hands down to feel his head and with the next contraction I pushed his lovely, warm, slippery little body out and he almost crawled up my tummy. . . . Although I had to have forceps we have a wonderful feeling of success.

First baby:

I did remember to look, and saw her head. I had steeled myself with stories of how disappointing new babies are but she looked perfectly beautiful!

First baby, very difficult operative delivery:

Mr B. arrived, examined me and took me straight into the operating theatre. I was completely happy as I trusted him absolutely and knew all would be well. I was anaesthetized so I don't know what happened next but my husband was there with me all the time and he saw his daughter born. . . . He talked to my husband the whole time explaining what was happening. My husband was the last person I saw before the anaesthetic took over and he was there as I woke to tell me that we had a little girl. I remember saying 'I love you both' before going straight off to sleep again! Although the baby wasn't able to come naturally in the end, it was a complete and incredibly wonderful experience for us both. C. was marvellous, and so gentle and calm all the time. I'm really looking forward to next time. I do feel that this is *our* baby as we shared her birth so completely. It's a wonderful, wonderful thing and we wouldn't have missed it for the world.

First baby:

My sensation was one of bursting at the seams (after an episiotomy). I could feel her head taking up the whole perineum. Crowning was quick and easy. After about 15 seconds Dr C. said, 'Push' and I saw her head. Dr C. suctioned the mucus from her mouth and she cried as I pushed the rest of her body out. After what seemed an eternity (one minute!) they brought little Katharine for me to hold. How happy and relaxed I felt! – lots of tears of joy. I only wish J. [her husband] could have been there too. A marvellous experience – I'd do it all over again tomorrow.

First baby:

They were prepared to do an episiotomy but I said I felt I could relax enough not to. By following the instructions of Sister L. when to push gently and when to pant the head was born without a

cut or tear. I was so excited and pleased that I was actually laughing
as the head was born. I could feel myself opening up. This was the
most thrilling moment as the head rotated and cried at once and
the body rushed out without waiting for another push. My husband
was delightedly exclaiming, 'Look, look, it's a boy.' We both felt
very pleased with ourselves. The staff were most kind and cooperative. They even brought my husband a cup of tea at 3 a.m. so
we could gloat over our feat together.

Second baby. P.O.P. spontaneous delivery:

I loved the feeling of the rest of the baby slithering out. . . . My
husband was with me all the time and Nurse N. thanked him for his
support afterwards. It was a great help having him there with his
arm behind my back especially when I had to push so long. He
kept reminding me of all sorts of things to help the breathing and
relaxing when I forgot towards the end.

First baby:

In what seemed a very short time I began to feel the birth outlet
stretching and then the midwife told me to be ready to pant with
the next contraction. I did this and felt the baby's head slide out.
I was all prepared to ask whether to push with the next contraction
when I heard the midwife instruct the student to 'lift the baby up
over the mother's abdomen' and with a sudden surge I felt the rest
of the body slip out. I had kept my eyes shut, being rather in-
timidated by the large audience, and quite forgot to open them as the
baby was born. Nevertheless it was a wonderful moment. I felt so
happy and excited it was some seconds before I thought to inquire
whether it was a boy or a girl. As soon as the cord was cut they
gave her to me to hold and my husband and I spent the next twenty
minutes gazing in admiration at our offspring. I can look back on
my labour as a very wonderful, though not painless, experience.

First baby:

I turned on my left side, the midwife said this would be easier for
delivery. Although I didn't know it at the time, she did an episiotomy and the head was born very soon after. It was thrilling:
I saw the rest of the baby being born with two more contractions
which came very easily, and although her first cry was a second or
two later, it seemed like hours. She had had the cord twice round
her neck, and it had to be cut after the head was delivered. Her

first cry was the most thrilling sound imaginable, the most welcome cry one can ever wish for. The nurse wrapped her in a blanket, and gave her to me, and the joy and happiness she gave to C. and me in just those few minutes was something which we shall treasure for ever.

Second baby, a posterior that rotated before delivery after a thirty-hour labour:

The head crowned and then slid out gently, and the baby began to breathe.... Any feelings of tiredness immediately vanished, and I think that I was the member of the group who was feeling fittest. I felt rather sorry for the doctor, when he turned up a few minutes later – there was nothing for him to do.

Second baby, after a traumatic first labour:

The midwife was just about to take her coat off and examine me when my stomach gave a lurch and I said I would have to push. In the rush to get the box open and a pad under me the baby's head crowned. As I was still asking whether I should push or pant I just had to push, and out came the head, twisted round as I watched it at a seemingly fantastic rate, and there was my son sliding out on to the bed like a rocket going into orbit! He announced his arrival with a fountain of water and a loud bellow, and the afterbirth slid out behind him. I have never experienced such happiness and joy, and such a sense of personal achievement.

First baby, P.O.P. spontaneous delivery:

My husband was with me the whole time and was a great comfort and help. He wiped my face with a cold flannel and reassured me that I was doing fine; both of these helped so much! The nurse told me to roll on my side – I didn't want to but she said I must as the babe was still facing the wrong way and it would be safer, so over I went, but what an effort. I felt glued to the bed! At the crowning I found panting helped when the nurse told me not to push – he crowned and yelled lustily and my husband announced that he had dark hair. I saw the rest of him born. He came very easily with one more gentle push. It was wonderful and I felt so clever! He weighed 8½ lb. My summing up of the whole thing was how well the word 'Labour' fitted. It was jolly hard work but well worth while. Nothing came as a surprise and I recognized each stage as it arrived and I felt quite happy the whole time.

AFTER THE BIRTH

The midwife begins to tidy up, while the mother who has been conscious and active throughout the birth and who has leaned forward to see her baby born is radiant and transfigured now. Far from feeling worn out, she experiences the glow of health and well-being and an overwhelming joy. She may feel that she has been enabled to share in the work of creation. She feels love for her husband who has been beside her and has helped her, so that they know that they have done this together, and a great spirit of thanksgiving.[1] As one new mother said, 'I feel swamped with love and affection for the world . . . It is because it was for me – and for H. [her husband] too – so complete an experience that I am so madly in love with the child.'

Sometimes there are other, less easily defined emotions – a slight regret that she cannot fall in love with the baby at one fell swoop, or a feeling of anti-climax. There is no need for her to pretend emotions she does not feel and she has earned the right to be honest about her emotions and to simply let things be as they are.

The midwife leaves and husband and wife are left alone with their child. Once they have proudly telephoned the grandparents they are suddenly aware of the peace of being together, the house quiet, with their sleeping child. They are now a family. They have experienced together something incomprehensibly wonderful – a peak of joy in their married life which will perhaps always be for them a symbol of the deepest sort of love they know. Their marriage has gained something from this – and through the months of pregnancy and the

1. Simone de Beauvoir, in *The Second Sex* (Cape, 1953), describes the feelings of a woman who must surely have been delivered under anaesthesia, so different are they from the experience of the woman who has had a natural birth. 'Some women suffer from the emptiness they now feel in their bodies: it seems to them that their treasure has been stolen. . . . But just what part has the mother had in the extraordinary event that brings into the world a new existence? She does not know. . . . There is an astonished melancholy in seeing him outside, cut off from her. And almost always disappointment.'

short space of a few hours in which new life entered the world it acquired a fullness of joy which, whatever their failings and mistakes later, can never be entirely forgotten. Such child-birth shared by husband and wife thus has a significance for both man and woman which reaches far beyond the act of birth itself, and through the family has its effect upon society as a whole.

CHAPTER 10

The Mother and Her Baby

THE CLOSENESS OF MOTHER AND BABY

WHEN her baby is born the mother naturally reaches out her arms to hold him. As soon as possible she likes to feel him close to her, nestling in the crook of her arm with his head on her breast. She looks at him with wonder and awe; can anything so perfect be born from her? This tiny, firm being has been cradled in her body for so long – she has known the child and yet not known him; they have learned together, both in pregnancy and in labour, the subtle rhythms of each other's bodies – but he was so indissolubly a part of her that she was unable to recognize him as a person distinct from herself. However fiercely possessive the mother may be in the first weeks after birth – and there is often a passionate tenderness in the way in which she wants to protect her child – the separation of the umbilical cord heralds the beginning of a separate existence, an individual life, for that child.

It is only because they are now distinct and separate beings and he is no longer rocked in the darkness of her body that the reciprocal relationship of love and need which finds its fullest expression in the experience of breast-feeding is possible. The baby begins to establish a relationship with the world through his mother. 'In the instinct to make contact (first by touch and then by visual "touch" of another being) the inborn *Thou* is very soon brought to its full powers, so that the instinct ever more clearly turns out to mean mutual relation, "tenderness".'[1] His first experiences of love and caring for another are given him in these times at the breast, and find their expression in bodily contact even before he is able to focus his eyes on his mother's face.

1. Martin Buber, *I and Thou* (trans. Ronald Gregor Smith), T. and T. Clark, 1937.

From the child's point of view (if he has one) birth may have come as a surprise, but we have little evidence to confirm or deny that it is in all cases traumatic and that it gives rise to the first anxiety, which forms a pattern for all later reactions to threat, as Otto Rank asserted. But if this is true the child who has been born naturally and easily is obviously at an advantage. A new-born child can have no conceptual understanding of its journey down the birth canal, but probably it is in a state of great neurological excitation. Its nervous system is suddenly flooded with stimuli with which it cannot cope and which must make its first impressions of the world 'a big, booming, buzzing confusion'.[1]

If the birth has been easy it is remarkable how soon the baby stops crying when his mother holds him, how soon the screams of protest are stilled, and with what willingness, as if returning to the breast rather than finding it for the first time, he suckles as he rests in the close haven of her arms.

The woman who is able to relax while holding her baby – and above all when feeding him – lets peace and contentment flow into him, and is less likely to encounter difficulties in the feeding relationship than the woman who cannot relax. Indeed relaxation is just as important after the baby comes as it was before.

First baby:

I haven't looked at a clock or thought about one side or the other and both Stephen and I are all the happier. The nurses are very nice about being a little flexible about times and so I feed him when he seems to want his feeds and we take just as long as he likes, and then after he is changed he seems to like just a few sucks more and then goes off to sleep.

First baby:

When I held the baby for the first time I don't think I experienced any rush of maternal feeling. That came in gradually, and then on about the fourth day after, it really hit me. It was like falling in love for the first time.

1. William James, *Principles of Psychology,* New York, 1890.

First baby:

Piers was obviously hungry, and just before visiting time, so I just said to the nurse, 'If you don't mind, I'm just going to draw my curtains and give the baby a few minutes at the breast to settle him down.' They were certainly sympathetic to my point of view, and we just quietly got on with it.

After a forceps delivery with general anaesthesia, first baby, deep transverse arrest:

I already am looking forward to the next pregnancy. In fact I can hardly wait. . . . I can't help but think about the wonder of it all. . . . After all, it is the biggest present a woman can ever give to the man she loves. It's strange but quite often I still feel an urge to give birth to my baby as though he is still in my womb.

SOME DIFFICULTIES

Sometimes if the birth has been long and difficult, or if the baby is premature and his nervous system not yet sufficiently mature to enable him to cope with the world, or if he has been doped with anaesthesia which the mother received during labour, and particularly if he has suffered a lack of oxygen, he starts off at a disadvantage, and feeding is no delight. The first need of both mother and baby after a difficult labour is obviously rest, but then the baby should be brought to the mother and should remain with her, for her to give him the love that is welling up in her and to fondle and stroke him as all babies should be fondled and stroked. Unless there are very serious and important reasons why the mother and child should be separated, and prematurity is not necessarily one of these, the mother should be free to create in those early days the close relationship of love and need which, it has been suggested by psychologists, is the basis for all satisfactory personality development. She will probably face difficulties in the feeding relationship; the baby may well prove apathetic and not want to feed, but she is being given a chance to know and observe her baby in a way that she can never do if he is isolated in a sterile hospital nursery. If she does not feel that in the space of ten or twenty minutes she has to get a certain number of ounces of milk into him, which is what often happens when the babies are brought to their mothers only at feeding times, she will not give way to despair. If the baby does not want to suck just then he can suck later, and perhaps he would prefer a number of small feeds to four or five large ones.

A good way of getting an apparently unresponsive baby to turn towards the breast and to grope for the nipple is gently and lightly to stroke the child's cheek nearest to the breast. A baby always turns towards a stroking movement at the side of the mouth. It does no good at all to push the baby's face towards the nipple, to open his mouth forcibly, to put glycerine or honey on the nipple or on to the baby's tongue, or to squirt milk into his mouth.

Whilst slapping a baby, tickling his feet or jogging him up and down may obviously achieve the result of waking him up at least temporarily, such activities are not likely to increase his appetite. The over-active, crying baby who seems to fight the breast, may be held firmly and calmly with great advantage,[1] but it is unlikely that battening his arms down in a tight shawl, fixing his head in a vice-like grip, and holding him as firmly encased as an Egyptian mummy will add to his content. Babies are not frightened by their arms waving in front of their faces, as some people believe. In fact, they very soon get rather interested in them and discover them as suitable playthings, so this is also no reason for swaddling a baby into a solid immobile bundle. Some babies scratch their faces badly, and the answer to that is to cut their fingernails rather than to tie their arms down.

Some mothers are concerned about the way in which their

1. An over-excited baby is best fed when still half asleep and certainly before he has had time to cry himself into a state of panic. Sometimes these babies are best lifted from the cot or pram still on the mattress, so that they are handled as little as possible before a feed. They may also like to be fed in a darkened room or, at any rate, away from bright lights. The mother of such a baby may find herself rocking as she feeds him or singing softly, and this is a spontaneous and often unconscious response to his need for a peaceful atmosphere. Each mother will learn for herself what is best for her baby.

new-born baby grunts, squeaks and sneezes, and lie awake that first night listening to noises and strange types of breathing which they feel sure are not natural. Although this can be alarming for the parents, it is quite normal and should not cause anxiety. A sneeze is a convenient way of clearing the nasal passages and young babies tend to sneeze a good deal.

Mothers may worry also about little sores on the baby's skin. The baby should be washed carefully and patted completely dry in all the creases of its body, especially in the area of the buttocks, behind the ears, in the folds of the neck, arms and legs, and between the fingers. A very little powder or cream can be smoothed on after the bath, but the skin must be bone dry before this is done or the child will very soon have caked lumps of talcum or grease in all the creases, which may result in open sores. Talcum powder or cream will also become sticky and unpleasant if the baby is allowed to become overheated or to cry until it is hot.

Bathing should be done in a leisurely way in a very warm room. Then there is no need for the mother to rush and to handle the baby hastily, and both can enjoy the process. *Everything should be prepared and at hand in advance* and the mother should be able to sit comfortably. Very little actual cleaning of the baby can be done when he is in the bath as the mother must concentrate on holding the slippery bundle: so the buttocks should be washed with an unscented soap and the folds and creases of the skin washed gently with small cotton wool swabs whilst he is lying on a big towel on his mother's lap before going into the water – eyes and face first, buttocks last, and a fresh swab for each area. The hair can be done next when necessary, by holding the baby's head over the bowl of water with his body wrapped up in the towel, using a small bowl of fresh water for rinsing.

Cotton-wool should not be left in contact with the buttocks, as it tends to cling and also to overheat the baby. Well rinsed muslin napkins which have had a blow in the fresh air or frequently changed disposable napkins are best against the baby's buttocks.

The hair should be brushed with a firm brush with rounded bristle-ends – not a very soft baby brush – and when it is washed the soap should be rinsed out very thoroughly or scurf may result.

Beyond this there is very little that a mother needs to know about care of the new baby, for his essential needs are for food and love. So the theme of this chapter continues to be that of breast-feeding and the intricacies and problems of the feeding relationship.

SUCCESSFUL BREAST-FEEDING

Breast-feeding can be quite painful during the first ten days or so, and no woman should be distressed if it proves not to be an unalloyed pleasure.

One of the difficulties that mothers often encounter in the early days is that of breast engorgement. Although painful *it is a good omen for successful breast-feeding*.

If a woman allows herself to become engorged when the milk first comes in, any time after the first twenty-four hours, she can suffer intense pain. The breasts fill up and become hot, tight and enormous. Rope-like knots stick out on the side of the breast under the arms, and the nipples recede under the surrounding inflamed mass so that the baby cannot get a grip on them. He must be able to get not only the nipple into his mouth, but also part of the areola (the brown area surrounding the nipple). Frequently ice-packs will cure this condition. Simply put cubes from the fridge into a nappy, and twist the ends. Tuck this inside the night dress, with towels around to absorb the drips.

If she has learned how to express colostrum during the later months of pregnancy, the mother will be able to express a little milk to ease the discomfort *immediately* she notices this state of affairs beginning. It is important to be able to do this herself, as it may occur in the middle of the night when no midwife is available to help her. Anyway, many women do not like their breasts being treated simply as milk-producing machines and do not want them touched by nurses if it can be avoided.

Holding the breast with one hand cupped under it, rhythmically press with the thumb and first finger of the other hand just above and just below the areola, and *think of the milk flowing*. Soon large drops of milk will begin to ooze out into the cup or washbasin. As you see it you begin to feel what seems like a great rush of milk from higher up in the *other* breast – the let-down reflex[1] – and a steady stream will pour out from the breast you are 'milking', bringing tremendous relief. You will probably not need to continue rhythmically pressing, as simple pressure on the breast will be sufficient for it to stream out in a great arc.

If you are unable to start the flow by simple expression in this way, you may need to massage the breast a little first. Holding one hand cupped under the breast, rub firmly with the palm of the other from side to side on the upper side of the breast. Then try expressing again. If still nothing happens and you are very uncomfortable, you may need gently to squeeze hot water over the breasts. Lean over a wash-basin or bowl and dipping a sponge into water as hot as you can comfortably bear pour water over and along the outside margin of the engorged breasts until milk drips steadily. You can then keep the milk flowing with steady pressure of the fingers of one hand, whilst supporting the breast with the other, until you are comfortable. Stop then, as over-expression will stimulate the breast to produce still more milk. If even this fails, a breast pump will relieve you if you ring up your doctor or midwife.

If at any time the nipples feel sore, keep them well oiled or creamed so that they remain supple; and if it is possible go back to nature and have a sun or air bath. A sun lamp can be used if one is *very* careful, but any part of the body not normally exposed tends to sun-burn easily. It is also important to protect

1. Stimulation from milking results in the release of oxytocic hormone from the posterior pituitary. This contracts the smooth muscle fibres of the small milk ducts, so forcing the milk into the big ducts, from whence it emerges through the nipple. See M. Newton and Niles Newton, 'The let-down reflex in human lactation', *Journal of Pediatrics* 33: 698, 1948. Niles Newton and M. Newton, 'Relation of the let-down reflex to ability to breast-feed', *Pediatrics* 5: 726, 1950.

one's eyes of course, and to have the baby in another room. Tell the midwife or doctor if the discomfort persists longer than a day. If the nipples are allowed to dry in the air or in the heat of the bulb from the bedside lamp during the first weeks of feeding the baby, the new mother will help to avoid any soreness.

If the breasts leak, and most women experience some leaking in at least the first six weeks or so, it is necessary to have turk-ish towelling pads inside the bra over the nipple. These can be bought shaped to the curve of the breast, but are rather expen-sive as one needs a change after each feed. Most of those on the market are waterproofed as well, but some women find that these hold the milk in against the breast too efficiently, and that the nipples tend to become very soggy and soft. In this case it is better to have only the towelling kind, except for parties or when dressed in one's best, and these can be copied in soft towelling if one buys a single pair as a model. Leaking from the breasts, incidentally, does not mean that a woman has too much milk. Washable dresses and blouses are best, and it is necessary to change the underclothes and bath frequently, or the breast-feeding woman soon smells like a cheesemarket. Gifts of good soap, bath salts and talc are greatly welcomed by the nursing mother. At least every day the mother will re-quire a clean bra and slip. A too tight bra or dress will press on the breasts so that, as they fill up towards feed times, milk may pour out. It is also necessary to change sheets and pillow-cases frequently, as when she is asleep the breasts may be pressing on the bed. She may not notice the smell, but it will probably be very unpleasant for her husband. In the days after the milk first comes in it may help to put an old towel underneath the top half of the body.

The new mother may wake early in the morning with the breasts very full and tender. If the baby is asleep, she should express some of the milk, and she may be able to get to sleep again for a little while. She should not make herself a pot of tea if the breasts are full like this, or she will become even more uncomfortable. This problem occurs not only in the first weeks but may also occur when the baby first decides to sleep through the night, but the milk supply will soon adjust to this.

Some lactation rituals of doubtful value

Most experts and baby books advise bathing the nipples with boiled water and cotton wool before and after feeding the baby, but I know of few women who do this, and it is one aspect of an over-evolved nipple culture in a society which is not noticeably successful in its breast-feeding practices.

Niles Newton, writing of the differences between markedly successful and unsuccessful breast-feeding, says:[1]

Successful breast-feeding is the type of feeding that is practised by the vast majority of mothers all over the world. It is a simple, easy process. When the baby is hungry, it is simply given a breast to suck. There is an abundance of milk, and the milk supply naturally adjusts itself to the child's growth and intake of other foods. It never occurs to the mother to worry about whether the baby is getting enough. The milk is ready and waiting to satisfy the baby's needs. Both mother and baby enjoy the process so much that weaning tends to be postponed rather than hastened.

Unsuccessful breast-feeding is a type of breast-feeding that is typical of the modern American urban mother. This type of breast feeding is a difficult and tenuous process. There is constant worry about whether there is enough milk for the baby. The mother is expected to regulate her diet, her sleep, and her habits of living to help make her milk good and plentiful. She worries about washing her nipples, and about which breast to give, and when and how long to give it. She often weighs the baby before and after feeding to see whether the baby has got enough, and is advised to express the milk remaining in her breast by hand after each feeding – a laborious process. Often the supply of milk is so insufficient that bottles must be resorted to to supplement the breast milk. Breast abscesses and engorgement, and nipple fissures and erosions frequently cause extreme pain. The pain, the work, and the worry of unsuccessful breast-feeding make early weaning part of the unsuccessful breast-feeding pattern.

It is for reasons such as these that we need to reassess the

1. *Maternal Emotions*, Hoeber, U.S.A. 1955.

value of the lactation rituals which are current in our society and see whether, in fact, they are helping or hindering us in the feeding relationship.

Mothers with a good milk supply need not feel that they must make efforts to empty the breasts, or at least one breast, with each feed, as many of the baby books assert. Some women find this a practical impossibility as the milk continues to flow, and if they change over breasts they feel the let-down reflex again in the other. It seems, therefore that 'complete emptying of the breasts', either by the baby alone or by the baby and by expression by hand afterwards, is not necessary and is only useful in those cases where the mother wishes to stimulate an inadequate milk supply.

One of the most dangerous of the doctrines which are at present accepted is that even though a mother is feeding 'on demand', breast-feeding should be regulated by the clock – that the baby should have so many minutes at one breast, and then be whipped over to the other side for so many further minutes, when the feeding experience is abruptly terminated, the child 'bubbled', cleaned up, changed and put down till next time.

But where both mother and baby love feeding times and have pleasure in their relationship each with the other, breast-feeding is not an isolated act reserved for certain set times of the day for a predetermined number of minutes. The child is not a car the tank of which has to be filled with petrol. Nor is it a dangerous animal which is to be thought of by those attending the mother as a little tyrant, gnawing at her nipples and draining away her strength.

The new-born child really is helpless. All his sensations are centred in his mouth, in the groping sensitive lips and tongue and here he finds his very first satisfactions.

> My Palate is a Touch-Stone fit
> To taste how Good Thou art.[1]

To separate him from his mother is to tear him away from the source of his life. He needs to feel his mother's loving care as

1. Thomas Traherne, 'The Estate', *Poetical Works,* Dobell, 1906.

she cuddles him and warms him with her own body, strokes his limbs and tiny fingers and the fine down on his cheeks, and as she responds to his quest for the sweet milk it is her privilege to give him.

It is a terrible thing for both the mother and the child to be deprived of these early satisfactions in their relationship – no less real for the mother than for her baby, and this is so whether the mother chooses to breast- or bottle-feed. But there may be reasons of maternal health as well why the mother able to feed her baby should do so.[1] It is almost incredible that people, because hospital regulations demand it, should believe it their duty to separate the mother and her baby and to break in on the developing relationship between them.

The mother wants to begin to know her baby and to have confidence in herself as a mother. The basis of all the faith she has in herself as a mother is laid then. She wants to be able quietly and in her own time, and without interference, to feel her way towards her child. She begins to learn that it is not enough even to love her baby; she must let him *know* by her warm bodily presence, flesh to flesh contacts and her answer to his need for cuddling and for milk, that she loves him. What does he like? What doesn't he like? Very often she wants to be completely alone when she feeds him so that she can experiment a little without feeling that she is likely to be criticized by the experts for her clumsiness of movement. She patiently observes her baby and discovers how he likes to be held and whether he minds her reading at the same time or wants her whole attention. She shifts her position so as to get more comfortable herself. She may want to discuss some of the techniques of feeding with an expert, and occasionally someone sitting quietly watching the mother feeding her baby can suggest certain changes in handling which can make feeding much

1. Breast-feeding appears to maintain breast health, and failure to breast-feed to predispose to the development of mammary cancer. See F. E. Adair, 'Etiological factors of mammary cancer in 200 women', *New York State Journal of Medicine*, 34: 61, 1934. H. J. Bagg, 'Experimental studies concerning the functional activity of the breast in relation to mammary carcinoma in mice', *Journal of Cancer Research*, 9: 498, 1925.

easier and pleasanter for both. But it is not the midwife's task to take businesslike command of the feeding situation, to put the nipple into the baby's mouth and hold him there, however desperately she wants to, however much she feels she could do it all so much better herself – and she should perhaps question the motivation of her own conduct in this respect. She may herself be longing to have a baby – and there is nothing unworthy in this. We hear a great deal in our society about sex drives, but little about a hunger which can be no less strong, and which may lead women to favour certain professions in which they are involved with the care of children – the hunger for motherhood.

BREAST- AND BOTTLE-FEEDING

The relationship of the child at the breast with his mother is not simply that of feeding, of getting nourishment – as any mothers knows. But books on baby-care, apart from an approving reference to the psychological benefits to the baby which are supposed to be derived from breast-feeding, rarely go into detail about the nature of the relationship, or about the psychological effects upon the mother.

We are told on the one hand that breast-feeding is important and desirable, and that it is our duty to feed our babies ourselves if we possibly can because breast milk is sterile (which it often is not), is just right for the baby, is at the right temperature, and gives him the comfort of our arms and our complete attention, and on the other hand, that it does not matter a bit if we cannot feed our babies ourselves because cow's milk and modern methods of artificial baby feeding – in the hands of an intelligent mother – are sterile and hygienic.

But of course breasts, fortunately, do not feel like bottles, and the communication of emotion by muscular tensions, by the plasticity of the nipple itself and by the actual flow of milk and other involuntary physical means is possible only when a baby is breast-fed. This is the great advantage that breast-feeding can have over artificial feeding, but conversely it obviously has certain disadvantages in a mother who is under stress, or for one reason or another feels that she cannot *give* milk to the baby.

One reason why some mothers dislike breast-feeding is that they feel that breast-feeding – and childbirth too – is something 'primitive', too elemental an experience for a civilized woman to be expected to enjoy.[1] Breast-feeding makes such a woman feel 'like a peasant' or 'a cow', degraded to an almost animal level of existence. The wording of some books giving advice on infant feeding does not always help; the reader is instructed to try and become cow-like – a particularly unfortunate simile when the woman, who may well have endured what she considers a humiliating experience during pregnancy and in the birth itself, is longing to be her former self again. One does not need to be particularly sensitive to dislike being compared to a cow. As we might expect, however, this feeling is rare among women who have prepared themselves for childbirth and who have found joy rather than degradation in the birth. But where it exists and is strongly felt it should be a contra-indication to breast-feeding, for this relationship is a personal matter, and if a woman has a resistance to it whilst at the same time struggling to do it because she feels she ought to, she may create many difficulties for herself and the child. If she could relax and enjoy feeding him with a bottle it would seem the obvious solution. After all, it is not so much *what* she feeds him with as *how* she feeds him that matters. It is her loving touch that he needs, and unsuccessful breast-feeding can be a very frustrating and disturbing experience for both mother and baby. Whilst breast-feeding can be the best sort of feeding there is, unsuccessful breast-feeding comes a poor second to happy bottle-feeding.

To some mothers breast-feeding is almost an erotic experience. 'The fusion sought in masculine arms – no sooner gran-

1. There are great cultural variations between different countries and social classes in this respect. Just after my first child was born a French Minister at a diplomatic dinner called across the table to me, 'And have you much milk for the baby?' – an unheard-of thing in Britain, which would have been positively shocking in the U.S.A., where in many hospitals women are given routine injections before birth in order to inhibit lactation.

ted than withdrawn – is realized by the mother when she feels her child heavy within her or when she clasps it to her swelling breasts. . . . The infant satisfies that aggressive eroticism which is not fully satisfied in the male embrace.'[1] They take frank delight in the feeling of the child at the breast and a few will speak openly of the intense pleasure it gives them.[2] I have known a mother turn away from a rather unsatisfactory husband and towards her baby in this way. Other women recognize the erotic element in breast-feeding and dislike it intensely. They do not wish to confuse what for them are two distinct levels of experience, the sexual and the maternal, and breast-feeding may be unpleasant for them for this reason. Dr Mavis Gunther[3] says that 'some consider it almost incestuous to offer the breast to the baby'. Still others, who are involved in some sort of psychological conflict the roots of which appear to lie in the marital relationship, do not want to feed their babies, or because they are seeking to withdraw from the relationship with their husbands as they know it, cannot wholly enter into the breast-feeding experience. Other women again cannot feel sexual delight as a result of stimulation of their breasts by their husbands while they are still feeding their babies. If they do not realize that this is quite a normal feeling they may get a little frightened. Some mothers indeed wonder whether childbirth has ruined their married life. G.P.s do not as a rule mention this subject in the brief discussions they have with their patients; midwives tend to find it embarrassing and irrelevant, and it is not the sort of subject which a young wife feels is grave enough to warrant going to an 'authority' for advice. It

1. Simone de Beauvoir, *The Second Sex*, Cape, 1953.
2. Breast-feeding – like sexual excitement – encourages uterine contractions, and hence, the rapid involution of the uterus to its non-pregnant state. Often mothers notice more severe 'after-pains' in the days following delivery when the baby is nursing. Women who have these contractions are more likely to be successful with breast-feeding than those who do not have them. See Chassar Moir, 'Recording the contractions of the human pregnant and non-pregnant uterus', *Transactions of the Obstetrics Society*, 54: 93, 1934; Niles Newton and M. Newton, 'Relation of the let-down reflex to ability to breast-feed', *Pediatrics*, 5: 726, 1950.
3. *Infant Feeding*, Methuen, 1970.

affects the husband too. Some men take direct delight in their wife's maternal functions and can enjoy the woman as a mother, feeling no resentment of the ten or eleven o'clock breast-feed at night. But many men cannot help feeling a little jealous of the baby then.

Understanding of the problem is certainly not a contra-indication to breast-feeding; it simply means that some adjust-ments are necessary.

We have seen that the child does not come to the breast only for food, and the technique of getting adequate nourishment is not the only thing he learns at the breast. His mother's arms form for him the centre of his universe. She is the giver and sustainer of life and from her touch comes all comfort and joy. It is tragic when a mother treats her child as an enemy, an invader who comes to suck her dry and tire her out and to take away her youth and attractiveness, leaving her weary and worn, only to scream and rage for more after a few hours and to batten on to her again like a leech. There is a John Bratby painting of a self-sacrificing Madonna in a state of complete physical exhaustion in an untidy kitchen cluttered with tins of infant food and other ritual implements for feeding a large, fat, muscular baby who is the Son whom she worships, the adored child before whom she lays her life. This is a not un-familiar scene in the homes of many conscientious mothers who feel themselves involved in a struggle with the baby. It is perhaps not so remarkable that under these circumstances advice is given to the mother to 'show the baby who is mas-ter', 'let him see you are in command'. But these are extra-ordinary words to use about this most tender and subtle form of human relationships, and hardly form an adequate response to the child's need for his mother and his adoration of her.

The child at the breast learns what it is to trust life.

But . . . the amount of trust derived from earliest infantile experience does not seem to depend on absolute quantities of food or demon-strations of love, but rather on the quality of the maternal relation-ship. Mothers create a sense of trust in their children by that kind of administration which in its quality combines sensitive care of the baby's individual needs and a firm sense of personal trustworthiness within the trusted framework of their culture's life style. This forms the basis in the child for a sense of identity which will later combine a sense of being 'all right', of being oneself, and of becoming what other people trust one will become.[1]

Ian Suttie sees the anxiety, hate and aggression which Freud believed to be primary instincts – built into human nature – and the drive for power which Adler believes to be a characteristic of human nature, as the pathological results of the refusal of the mother to give to the child or her withdrawal from the child when he still needs her, and when her absence results in terrifying loneliness and loss of security. Aggression, he says, is not a spontaneous emotion. The good mother is the warm, responsive mother, the mother who is there when the child needs her, the mother who does not deny her feelings of tenderness towards the child, and who can express these feelings, who kisses and cuddles and handles the baby with spontaneous affection. (There are women who are 'frigid' with their children, or with one particular child, no less than there are women who are frigid with their husbands.) It is not that aggression is in the baby from birth waiting to burst out. It grows out of the mother-child relationship, and when a child is abnormally aggressive something has happened between mother and baby which resulted in the mother emotionally rejecting the child or the child being afraid that the mother will reject him.

Our adult, grudging, materialistic minds have decided that the baby gets the best of the partnership with the mother, and we talk of the mother's 'sacrifice'. The mother-child relationship, however, (to the child's mind) is a true 'balanced', symbiosis; and the *need to give* is as vital, therefore, as the *need to get*.[2]

PLAY AT THE BREAST

One of the most important experiences that the child at the breast can have is that of *play*. However hasty a woman, and

1. Erik Erikson, *Childhood and Society*, Penguin, 1965.
2. Ian Suttie, *The Origins of Love and Hate*, Kegan Paul, 1935.

however efficient she considers herself to be, she should realize that the baby is not there just to suck like a machine. First of all, the child will play only with his lips and tongue, and only later will he learn the pleasure of stroking her breast or the stuff of her petticoat or dress with his fingers and the palm of his hand, or of 'bouncing' or bumping her breast, or even pounding, and enjoying its elasticity and texture.

At first his keenest delights are situated in the area of the mouth and from even the very first weeks of pleasurable sucking he may try licking, pecking, rolling the nipple between his lips, nibbling and making small plosive movements of the lips against the sides of the breast if he is allowed to nestle in and play with his mother's body. There is nothing shocking or 'unhealthy' about this, even though midwives tend to frown upon this playing at feeding and to fear that the mother will end up with painfully sore nipples. The baby who makes nipples sore is the one who battens on to the breast when he comes to his mother, urgently hungry and clamouring – not the one who can casually play with his mother whenever he feels like it and who feels the closeness of her flesh when the satisfaction of hunger is not immediately necessary.

PLANNING ONE'S DAY

It is true that to achieve this sort of relationship with her baby the mother must organize her day around the baby rather than struggle to fit the baby in with some preconceived routine suggested by an outsider or worked out from a book. The baby must come first. Hard as this may sound, once one has agreed to establish this relaxed attitude towards housework and domestic routines – and to those extra-domestic activities which the mother may, quite rightly, be trying to perform – it becomes easier rather than more difficult to evolve a routine which fits in approximately with the baby's need for attention. The new-born baby has a pattern of sleeping, eating and nuzzling play, of which one only has to become aware before one can guess roughly the most convenient times to wash the nappies or bake a cake or to run out to the shops. It is the mother who is fighting her baby and getting more and more tense while she listens to him scream, who finds the greatest difficulty in finding time to do things and in creating a peaceful and happy atmosphere in the home for her husband. In dealing with a tiny baby, the easiest way for all concerned is to omit all 'shoulds' from one's thinking and to allow oneself to enjoy the baby just as he is.

Human beings are more important than the uncleaned fire-place and the unwashed-up dishes, and it does not really matter what other people think. If it does matter to the mother, she can always keep one room clean and tidy so that she knows she has somewhere to welcome visitors and to give the appear-ance of a well regulated household.

Even a baby's physical health can be as, or even more, dependent upon tender loving care than it is upon hygienic surroundings. In the classical study made by Rene Spitz,[1] out of ninety-one babies in a Foundling Home who were given every physical attention, whose diet was carefully planned and whom 'no person whose clothes and hands were not steril-ized' could approach, but who were deprived of maternal affection or any substitute for it – thirty-four died, and most of the remainder were severely retarded in development. In the control group of illegitimate children left with their mothers – many of them uneducated working girls – the babies develop-ed normally and not one died.

The day's routine is largely determined by when the new-born baby wants to eat, and it is easiest for mother and baby to like each other if the child is fed 'on demand', at any rate in the first weeks. Gradually the mother will perceive that the baby can bear to wait for his food a little, and as the mother begins to take up the threads of a wider social life and activities outside the home she can adjust the feeds a little to suit her convenience, unless this should prove to make the baby very unhappy, in which case he is not yet ready for it. No baby should ever be left to scream with rage and fright; small babies are not 'naughty' when they cry. They are either in pain or

[1] 'Anaclitic Depression', *The Psychoanalytic Study of the Child,* vol. II. International Universities Press, 1946.

they are frightened or frustrated. The baby does not yet know that the mother's whole day is so organized as to give him food, warmth, dry clean napkins, and cuddling. To him his universe is still totally unorganized and shadowy. After some weeks he begins to trace the pattern and to expect definite activities. When his mother picks him up and cradles him in her arms in the way he knows, he is going to be fed. When he hears the water rushing and smells the comfortable scent of towels airing in front of the fire, it is going to be bath-time. Gradually he begins to appreciate the security of an approximately mapped day.

But we can imagine that to the new baby hunger is a terrifying experience. Not only is it painful, but he has no knowledge that the torture will ever cease. Adults smile with amused tolerance as his wail rises in a crescendo of fury but those who are capable of imaginatively reliving this experience of early babyhood will not smile. For the child is in terror. He knows nothing but his desire. He feels completely isolated and lost.

The baby cannot distinguish between 'me' and 'not-me'; his own sensations are his world, *the* world to him; so when he is cold, hungry or lonely there is no milk, no well-being or pleasure in the world – the valuable things in life have vanished. And when he is tortured with desire or anger, with uncontrollable, suffocating screaming, and painful, burning evacuations, the whole of his world is one of suffering; it is scalded, torn and racked too.[1]

Books on baby-care, weighing the child regularly, even test weighing before and after feeds, cannot tell a mother when her baby is hungry. Only the baby himself can do that. *Before the child begins to learn from his mother the mother must learn from the baby*.

There is one safe rule for every new mother to follow: *if a new-born baby cries it almost invariably wants to be fed*. It is as simple as that. The apocryphal safety pin stuck in its bottom which one reads about in all the baby books is most unlikely to be the cause. It is highly probable that the child is hungry.

1. Joan Riviere, *Love, Hate and Aggression*, Hogarth Press, 1962.

Occasionally a rather excitable baby is perfectly contented to be picked up and carried around, or rocked, or just nestled in one's arms, where he can hear the steady heart-beat which accompanied his intra-uterine existence. My first four babies did not want this and were happy to be put down when they had dropped off to sleep at the breast. I thought it was because I knew how to handle my babies. I was wrong. My fifth baby was sociable from the start, and particularly wakeful in the evenings. Such are the comments of other mothers and older women that a woman feels rather guilty at letting a baby stay up. There is nothing wrong with it, if you can stand it, and at about three months the baby will begin to conform to a more 'normal' routine. It is much better to accept that that is the kind of baby you have than to try and fight it.

At about three months a small inclined seat which can be stood on the draining board or the table or wherever the mother is working can be extremely useful, and a little later still a bouncer, of which there are several on the market, is invaluable if it is suspended where the child can watch the mother at her chores, well away from hot water, kettles, knives and electric plugs and flexes!

COMPLEMENTING BREAST-FEEDS

If the baby is wakeful and ill at ease between feeds, or if he seems not to be growing, getting fatter and bigger and 'filling out', you can try the effect of giving him extra food by 'topping up' with cow's milk *after* breast-feeds. This would seem to be such an obvious course of action that it is unnecessary to state it, but it is surprising how many mothers feel that they must choose between breast-feeding and bottle-feeding exclusively and that the combined method involves too much hard work. Some babies like to be topped up after the late-afternoon feed only, when the mother may be rather weary and not able to give the baby as much as at earlier feeds of the day. There is nothing shameful about this.

The milk for topping-up can be prepared before the breast-feed in bottle, cup or even wine glass. The baby can suck it or drink it from a spoon or from a narrow-rimmed glass or cup. A number of small babies cannot easily tolerate very rich milk, so it is as well to dilute it slightly. They also like it sweetened. Until the baby is several months old the milk should be boiled even though it is pasteurized.

Except in very hot weather, it is unlikely that the baby will require extra drinking water.

It is not necessary to drink excessive quantities of liquid if one is breast-feeding. A mother should drink just as much as she wants. Many women feel thirsty as the milk flows, and like to drink at the same time as the baby. If it is a hot drink the mother must be ready for the first day when the baby lashes out with his fist when she least expects it, and knocks the cup over. Once a baby is kicking and waving his arms around it is unwise ever to drink hot liquid with him in her arms, or to allow anyone else to do so.

ENCOURAGING THE MILK SUPPLY

The best thing that mothers can do to encourage their breast-milk is to bask in the sun all day and be cosseted and pampered by a loving husband, but since both sun and, on occasion, the loving husband may be absent, and since the mother probably finds herself busier than ever before, she must seek other ways of increasing her milk supply if she fears that she has not enough to satisfy the demand.

The more stimulation the breasts are given by the baby's sucking, the more likely are they to respond by producing milk. A hungry baby wants to be fed more often, and in this way the supply is soon increased. Demand regulates supply quite naturally. It is not necessary to have a single clock in the house in order to be able to breast-feed a baby satisfactorily. There is no need to look at the time or to work out how long he has gone between feeds or to note down how many times the mother has fed him in the last twenty-four hours, even though she will be constantly asked the last question. The practice of timing the duration of breast-feeds is dangerous, because the mother has her eye on the watch instead of the baby, and is not concentrating on giving the milk and the pleasure of its flow as she might be if she were not so uncertain of herself and lacking in confidence. She can shift the baby over from one breast to the other side when his rate of swallow to suck slows down, i.e. when he has to press the nipple more often before he swallows a mouthful, or when he begins to look around and get interested in other things. A mother does not actually need to observe this phenomenon consciously; she just feels that it is time to change over, and unconsciously reacts to the change of rhythm. Then she lets him go on at the second breast as long as he wants. When he begins to play around she spends a little longer enjoying him, letting him play with the breast, and then changes him.

Whilst a baby still minds waiting for food it is best to change him after feeds, or at any rate after he has had one side, rather than before, and also better to bath him after a feed if the mother can do it without bouncing him about too much and making him sick. Babies vary greatly in the ease with which they bring back food, but the mother can help by learning the technique of undressing, bathing and dressing the baby again without unnecessary movements. Ideally she should only have to turn the baby over once when undressing him, but this rather depends on the sort of clothing he wears. It is useful to have neck openings wide enough to enable the clothes to be slipped on over the legs, or to have cross-over or envelope neck openings. The technique of undressing and bathing can be learned at mothercraft classes before the baby comes, or from the midwife afterwards.

In order to get the rest she requires, it is a good idea for the mother to make a habit of feeding the baby on a bed or couch with her feet up, making herself really comfortable and luxurious if possible, with a blanket or rug, a hot water bottle if she is cold, a drink and a book. A divan downstairs can be of great use, as there are numbers of household tasks which can be done lying on a bed.

When things seem to be getting on top of her — and at times they are bound to — she should drop everything as soon

as possible and take to her bed for a rest. Ten minutes of relaxation and peace then is better than hours of it later when she
has let herself begin to feel really weary and ill.

MUSCULAR REHABILITATION

The midwife will give the new mother a list of exercises for
her to do, or if she is in hospital the physiotherapist will come
round to teach newly delivered mothers suitable exercises for
the puerperium (the six weeks following childbirth). These are
usually started the day after delivery, and are graduated so as
to exercise the muscles without straining them. A woman will
already have done some exercises during pregnancy which will
be helpful now.

. One of the most important exercises is to tense the muscles
of the pelvic floor. The contraction of these muscles is now
more important than their relaxation. If a woman has had
stitches she may not be able to do this at first as it can be painful, but she should do it as soon as it does not hurt. However it
is important to consider this not only as an exercise for set
times of the day, although in order to ensure that she does not
forget it, it is a good idea to do it every time she washes up
and when she feeds the baby – but to cultivate a habit of holding
these muscles firm. With well-prepared muscles during pregnancy, a controlled second stage, without unnecessary forcing
and straining, and carefully exercised muscles during the
weeks that follow, a woman can be as small and tight inside
as before she conceived her baby, and instead of taking a larger
contraceptive diaphragm, for example, she may discover that
she needs to be fitted with the identical size.

THE MOTHER'S DIET

During the puerperium many women find that they get constipated and it is customary for midwives to advise dosing
with laxatives on the third or fourth day after the birth. Strictly
speaking this should not be necessary, and with early ambulation and post-natal exercises which give massage of the ab-

domen, often all that is necessary is that the new mother should have raw fruit, plenty of 'roughage' including porridge and bran and, if she wishes, some laxative foods such as stewed prunes or figs. All straining on the lavatory should be avoided, as this can cause stress to an already stretched pelvic floor.

The nursing mother need not feel that she must worry about her diet all the time she is feeding her baby. It is not necessary to eat excessively large quantities of protein in the form of meat and fish in order to feed a baby, although she may find that she likes to drink more milk. However, large quantities of milk are not essential in order to produce milk; a cow does not herself drink milk. Many vegetarians find no difficulty in breast-feeding.[1] If the mother wishes to get her weight down she should concentrate on fresh fruit, vegetables and salads, and cut down on carbohydrates, as any magazine article on slimming will tell her. If she gets hungry between meals she may like eating cheese in blocks like chocolate.

NURSERY MATTERS

The mother is bound to be given much good advice by nearly everyone she comes into contact with – friends, relations, people in shops, the daily help, women who have never had a baby, and above all her mother. One would feel tremendously isolated as the mother of a first baby without all this advice pouring in, and it is a sign of people's love for small helpless babies and their longing to do something about it. If one realizes this one can receive even the most officious of instructions with a good grace.

The baby must be allowed to cry and the mother must get some rest, she will be told, for if the child does not cry 'his lungs won't expand'. But a mother is rarely able to rest while her baby is crying, and should not try to. If she wants to lie down she can take him with her into bed. The baby's lungs will expand all right anyway.

She must eat certain foods she heartily dislikes or her milk

1. The author herself, who is a vegetarian, breast-fed her twins for nine and a half months without strain or deterioration in health.

will go. Unless baby wears woollen booties, bonnet and gloves she will almost certainly be told that he is cold, and people will worriedly feel his hands and feet. He must not lie on his front or he will smother himself. He ought to be weighed, given gripe water, extra vitamins, Virol, magnesia, water between feeds, cereal, pip and peel water – all of these and more may be suggested.

The simpler the baby's clothes are, the better. The easiest is to have all the openings either at the front or at the back so that dressing and undressing becomes a simple operation. Long strings and ties are best avoided as the baby soon starts sucking these. Unless it is windy the child is unlikely to require a hat. Booties always get kicked off and lost as soon as the child is moving at all, and mittens stop him from exploring his fingers. They will also get sucked and very dirty.

Vests should be silk and wool or cotton rather than pure wool in the first months as babies' skins are often very sensitive to irritation. The mother may find that he gets a rash under his chin from the wool of the matinee coat and that she has to put something like a soft bib or some cotton over it.

Vest, nappy, open-leg-style plastic knickers, night-gown and coat or all-in-one baby-suit should be sufficient, with warm shawls or blankets for snuggling him in and for carrying him from room to room. As soon as he begins to kick he should have warm, capacious baby-bags.

To feel if a baby is warm enough, the mother can touch him at the back of the neck, where he should feel comfortably warm. If she is not sure, she should feel his tummy and back. Although babies should not be permitted to go blue with cold, it stands to reason that neither should they be bright pink with heat.

Some mothers are not sure of the position in which the baby should sleep. The mother can put the baby down in any way she likes provided that he does not have a pillow. Even very tiny babies can turn their heads from left to right and adjust their position if they are put on their fronts, so if she likes her baby to have some choice in the matter himself she may prefer to lay him down on his front, with his head to one side, in the American way. A baby brings up bubbles of wind rather more easily lying in this position than lying on his back and is less likely to inhale vomited milk, but it may be necessary to change the cot sheet more frequently. One disadvantage of this method is that other people will think the baby is smothered and in the mother's absence may wake him up.

Weighing can be of little positive help to mother or baby, and the time is better spent in cuddling and playing. Only if the baby is ill (or if the mother thinks he may be) is there some point to it.

A breast-fed baby under three months old is unlikely to need any extras. Even after that age it is unlikely that he will require anything else until the mother feels that he is old enough to begin to explore different tastes. It is the mother who feels very uncertain of herself and who feels that she cannot possibly be producing good milk for her baby who starts stuffing the child with other things. This may do good if it restores the mother's confidence, and if giving the baby a daily dose of milk of magnesia makes a woman feel a good mother she can do so. But it is for the mother's rather than for the baby's benefit that it is done. After about six weeks she can start cod liver oil (or vitamin A and D drops if the baby does not like it), and a vitamin C-rich juice, but she should not make a ritual even of this. The baby will probably flourish without it.

If a woman enjoys feeding her baby, she should use her own feelings and the baby's capacity for enjoying new experiences of this kind as guides as to when to start weaning him. There is no need to follow the text book. All she needs to remember is to introduce new tastes gradually and to cut out anything that he does not like. She can start introducing new tastes from a few weeks old if she wants to, but this is likely to mean more work for her. If she thinks of weaning as introducing new flavours rather than as cutting out breast-milk she will find that there will be no abrupt transition, and no weaning 'crisis'. So many people treat weaning as taking something *away* from the baby that it still wants, but it is rather a question of *enlarging the child's experience*. When he really likes other foods he will enjoy having them before the breast-feed and then will tend to take less of her milk after. Until that time, it is best to feed him first and give him a taste or two of finely grated apple or cereal or what the mother will after he has satisfied his immediate hunger.

There is no need for a baby to have a bottle at all, although it is as well to have one in the house, and if the mother wants to leave him in the care of others for short periods it is helpful if he is accustomed to the idea of milk coming in a bottle in case of emergency. He can be started on a cup as soon as the mother wants to give him tastes of cow's milk. Babies very soon get interested in what their mothers are eating and drinking and enjoy bits and pieces off her plate and sips from a cup on her tray.

Cutting out a breast-feed entirely will probably mean that the milk supply will become less, not more, so if a mother wants to continue breast-feeding her baby, she should give him some breast milk with each feed.

Despite theory to the contrary, experience has taught some mothers that protest at weaning is not inevitable. It is possible to allow a baby to wean himself by observing his wishes carefully. The prerequisite to this is that the mother represents the world as an exciting place and that eating is fun for them both. It may help if both mother and baby eat at the same time. There is no magic about nine months old that means that the mother must drop the last breast-feed just then and that there is something wrong in continuing to feed her baby longer. Many babies enjoy sucking for some weeks or months more, and some are ready to drop it earlier. If for her own convenience it is important to finish breast-feeding, she should let the child enjoy a bottle as long as he will.

When a child of nine months or older is picked up for a breast-feed and reaches out for the milk jug on mother's tray, quite obviously preferring it to his mother's milk, it is time to drop the last breast-feed. However this does not mean that from that hour henceforward he should be banished from the breast. It may be that later in the day he starts missing that time with her, and if he seems miserable, she should feed him. He may still like to cuddle into her breast occasionally, even though there is no milk or he does not want food, and it suggests an unnecessarily puritan conscience to deny him this pleasure.

AN EVOLVING RELATIONSHIP

As a baby gets older he will be able to wait for a feed without becoming desperate, and will enjoy filling in the time watching branches of trees in the wind, leaves fluttering, grasses shaking, shadows moving, people passing, curtains at the window or washing on the line. The mother who knows her child well will see when this stage has been reached and will gradually begin to free herself from her close bondage with the newborn child. From the moment that the child was born the two have begun to grow away from each other, and now a second landmark is reached. The child no longer needs her so insistently and urgently; he starts to turn towards the world and its wonders. However strong mother-love is, and however possessive in the first weeks of the child's life, the relationship must evolve. I have stressed the closeness of the mother–child relationship; it is also necessary to emphasize that it is a living, growing relation, and its richest reward is found in its fruition in adult poise and independence. The child cannot remain bound to the mother. The mother must know when to draw the child towards her and when to let go, and this involves a delicate sense of timing not only during adolescence but even in the first months of life.

CHAPTER II

The Parents' Adjustments

PSYCHOLOGICALLY, the first months after the birth of the first child are a time in which great adjustments are necessary. The mother – even though she hesitates to admit it – often harbours a secret resentment against the baby who has deprived her of her freedom and the leisure of bachelor-girl life which continues in a modified form for the first year or so after marriage, until the birth of the first child. Now she may have no money of her own, no personal allowance and no joint bank account with her husband, and has to squeeze money for her clothes, her personal luxuries (if she has any) and presents from the housekeeping money. She feels tied down by maternity and domesticity. She struggles with tasks for which she has not been trained and which recur day after day with monotonous regularity. She longs to be again the carefree girl she once was, and this desire makes her feel guilty and adds further to the strain.

The baby, too, will almost certainly prove exasperating at times, and even when he is still tiny and she thinks she 'should' be having only sweet and loving feelings about him, she may be shocked to discover that she hates him as well as loving him. Babies are not always very cooperative, and just when we have planned to go out or are dressing up for a party they demand our attention.

DISAPPOINTMENT WITH THE BABY

Although most mothers can face up to their emotions of anger and irritation at such times, it is less easy to admit that one is disappointed in the baby, that one imagined that somehow he would be very different and altogether more like one's mental picture of an 'ideal' baby.

During pregnancy and after the announcement of the birth

the young mother is bombarded with baby books, advertisements and photographs of babies obviously bursting with health and merriment, taken from just the angle at which they look their most roguish and charming. She looks at her own baby, who probably has a rash on his cheek, a sore behind his ear, a receding chin, a blister on his lips from hard sucking, eyes that do not yet focus on anything and skin that seems very pale beside that of these rosy-cheeked babies. What has she produced, she wonders? She feels guilty – first because she must be a bad mother because her child does not look like the pin-up babies, and secondly because she feels awful at preferring the look of the advertisement baby to the real live one in her arms. Other mothers visit her with their babies, weeks or months older, who have survived these rashes, sores and other disfigurements and are usually extremely attractive, intelligent and bonny. These mothers rarely mention that their children too looked very much like that when they were three weeks old. They give conflicting kinds of advice, and depart to discuss, the mother feels sure, the disadvantages of her baby as compared with theirs. Yes, they probably do; such is mother love.

Hard as it is, the mother should relax, laugh at her earnestness, and enjoy her baby for what he is, just as he is, at this stage of his young life. That is the beginning of knowing and loving her baby *as a person*. She should tell the health visitor of her worries about his skin and his scalp, and all the other things that are on her mind. But above all, she must accept her baby in his individuality, for himself. In a few weeks time he will look much more like the magazine advertisements.

This sort of stress may be of particular importance in relation to the mother's ability and skill in breast-feeding her baby. She becomes over-concerned or anxious and concentrates all the resources of her mind on a task which is essentially one of spontaneous mothering. Or she does not want to feel so tied to the baby, and yet society tells her, in many different ways and through varying media, that this is expected of her, and that she is harming her baby if she will not give him the special cherishing of feeding him herself. But she wants to keep her milk. She wants her breasts to be her own and not to belong to the baby.

And, often dimly aware of this, she worries that she does not love her baby, this strange little animal in whom she has a detached but protective interest. Such women need reassurance that more developed feelings of affection will quickly grow as they get to know their babies better. And it is important that they should not feel confined to the home or shut off from their former friends.

THE HUSBAND'S JEALOUSY OF THE CHILD

The mother's secret resentment of the baby can be further exaggerated by the husband's jealousy of his child, or this may present a problem of its own. The husband dislikes the baby or is simply not interested in him. (The baby is often a boy in these cases. The father points out to the mother that their son is ugly, that he does not, yet at any rate, show any obvious signs of intelligence, that he wails at inconvenient times, and that she is at his beck and call instead of at her husband's.)

These signs of resentment of the child tend to be the exception rather than the rule in cases where the husband has been needed during his wife's pregnancy and has helped her actively in labour. Instead of feeling that the baby has usurped his rightful place, he thinks of him as something he has helped to create, not merely by impregnation but also by the care, loving attention and moral support he has been able to give his wife during the months of her preparation for childbirth and the birth itself. The husband who has been of active assistance to his wife – who may have seen the wrinkled crown of the baby's head even before she did – and whose arms were perhaps the first in which the new-born child was laid, is unlikely to be under the misapprehension that he was unnecessary and superfluous.

But where the husband is left to pace the floor during the birth and is treated afterwards as a dangerous carrier of microbes threatening the health of his wife and baby, it is not surprising that he may feel jealous of the baby, and unwanted. There is a tendency for the doctor and midwife, even in the home situation, to treat the husband as a liability. He is crowded out of the way by the midwife, the G.P., the home-help, the health visitor, the grandparents, other relatives and women friends, and the new baby reigns as the centre of attention of all these solicitous invaders of the home. This is further accentuated by the non-permissive attitude of doctor and midwife towards the resumption of sexual relations. The husband must leave his wife strictly alone apart from bringing her cups of tea and bunches of flowers. The midwife may demand that the husband should sleep in a separate bed, or even in another room.

Under these circumstances, a woman should not be shocked if her husband harbours some jealousy of the baby. He is usually unwilling to recognize this jealousy and will not admit it if she questions him about it directly. But she should not allow herself to become indignant about it. The isolation he feels from his wife, whom he has had to himself up to now, may be further exacerbated by childhood experiences of am-bivalence towards a younger sibling with which he never came to terms. He needs to be reassured that he is still loved and wanted and that he is a wonderful husband and father.

SOME WAYS IN WHICH THE HUSBAND CAN HELP

It is important that the husband should back his wife up in all that she is trying to do and should act to a certain extent as a buffer between her and criticism coming from those outside the home. A pregnant woman is highly vulnerable to warnings and criticism coming from older women, and above all to advice emanating from her own mother, who may be anxious and worried about her. Once the baby is born it is necessary for the husband to reassure his parents that he has perfect confidence in his wife's ability as a mother and that he stands by her in the way in which she is attempting to bring up her child. If the husband starts criticizing the wife's efforts and helps to make her feel a failure, she may soon stop trying, and caring for the baby will degenerate into a series of wearisome chores. The best way for him to help is to tell her that she is a marvellous mother. All the work seems worth while then.

If the husband can develop his domestic skills in dealing with the baby so that he can give his wife a rest occasionally, so much the better. This comes easily to some fathers, who thoroughly enjoy themselves changing nappies and bathing their offspring, but it is very hard on others.

DEPRESSION

Sometimes, however, the new mother goes through a black patch which does not seem to lift, and feels a despair which seems out of all proportion to the problems presenting themselves. There may be difficulties in feeding the baby, or in getting enough sleep, but most women prove fairly resilient, and given just one good night's sleep or a satisfactory feeding time, quickly bounce back into cheerfulness. But some do not – and cannot – however much they may feel they ought to, and however much they are told, cruelly, to 'snap out of it' or pull themselves together.

The mother suffering from puerperal depression often resents the baby and its demands on her, may find it is not the baby she really wanted (not pretty, or big enough, or neat and small enough, or not a boy, or not a girl) and frequently becomes completely disinterested in it, retiring to bed, or sitting blankly staring at the wall, withdrawing completely from the problems which seem insuperable. Even though people come in to help, and even though her husband stays home to do the housework and cook, which sometimes happens, her real problems are still with her, of course, because they are problems inside herself.

Depression usually suggests a mental state in which one is miserable, and because being sad may not be the most obvious thing about postnatal depressive illness, it may seem a misnomer for a state in which a woman ignores and neglects her baby, or wants to kill it, or is convinced that it has died – or in which there simply seems to be no continuity of experience between herself during pregnancy and the woman she is now. But this is what it is. She may also have times when she is confused and disoriented, not knowing exactly where she is or whether it is day or night, and may attempt suicide. It is obvious that this is mental illness, and that skilled help, drugs and psychotherapy are probably needed. The husband should not wait for his wife to agree to go to the doctor, but should go himself if she will not come, and ask the doctor to visit, and whether he feels it desirable to get psychiatric help. Madness can be a terrifying thing, and a woman can put off seeking help – either because of a total inertia, or because she or her husband are ashamed to acknowledge the need for expert guidance. There is no reason to think that given help of this kind a woman may not, after a few months to sometimes a year or so, again be living a useful and positive life.

If you feel depressed the chances are that you are *not* embarked on a mental illness, but that it is an emotional 'growing pain'. However well-organized and placid other women seem, most suffer the same doubts and worries. There is no quick remedy – no miracle drug – for the suffering that is the necessary accompaniment of growing up; stress produces a challenge, and an opportunity for fresh resources. Having a baby is an important time when such new adjustments need to be made.

SEXUAL RELATIONS AFTER THE BABY COMES

After the baby is born, a couple can make love whenever they feel drawn together, but it is wise to wait for complete intercourse until the period during which the woman is losing a blood-stained discharge is over. It is quite normal for this to last from about five days when the involution of the uterus is very rapid to about three weeks in cases when it is taking place more slowly. Often the discharge appears to have stopped, but is noticed again on getting up in the morning or after breast-feeding the baby.

To some women erotic excitement does not return very quickly after childbirth, and especially is this likely to be so if they feel sore or tender as a result of the birth. Although it is quite possible for a woman who has had a natural birth to want intercourse three or four days afterwards, it is usually ten to fourteen days or longer before desire is aroused. It is important for the husband to prepare the way with words and not to rely upon direct physical stimulation alone. Some men think that women are not so responsive to words as they are themselves. A man may neglect to say the things that once he said when he was first discovering the delights of the woman's mysterious body, and approached her in wonder and reverence – 'with my body I thee worship'. Although words may not have the same direct effect upon the genital organs in women as they can have in men, and it is unlikely that a woman can be roused in this way to the same heights of sexual pleasure as a man when he has an erection as a result of words alone, loving words can pave the way towards physical excitement. Love-play after childbirth should always be initiated by tenderly-spoken, loving words. After a woman has borne a child she wants to be told that she is still lovely in a man's eyes and that her naked body can still rouse him to desire. She does not want to be just a maternal figure, and she fears sometimes that she has bartered the romantic side of their love for the privilege of children, and for becoming a sort of fertility symbol, a goddess of abundance.

A woman wants to be assured that her girlhood is not suddenly incalculably far behind her, and if it is her first child, and especially if it was conceived early in marriage, she wants to feel that the love of pre-marriage and newly married days has not changed. In any marriage in which the love relationship develops it does change, of course, and should be richer and fuller as the years go by, but this is very difficult for the new mother to accept. She would rather find again the love she knew than be expected to adapt herself to a love which, though it may be more mature, she fears is devoid of the romantic and mysterious elements, the pleasant shock of discovery of each other, and the thrill of a touch which reveals hidden emotions and new desires.

A newly married couple, passionately in love with each

other, cannot believe that their love will ever change, or if it does, are convinced that this must be to something much more lukewarm, something altogether inferior:

> That time when all is over, and
> Hand never flinches, brushing hand;
> And blood lies quiet, for all you're near;
> And it's but spoken words we hear,
> Where trumpets sang; when the mere skies
> Are stranger and nobler than your eyes;
> And flesh is flesh, was flame before;
> And infinite hungers leap no more
> In the chance swaying of your dress;
> And love has changed to kindliness.[1]

After the first baby has been born to them, it is the husband's responsibility to reaffirm his desire for the woman's body and his adoration of her as a bride.

The woman may find after the baby is born that she is rather slower for a time in responding fully to her husband's desire for her, and that she cannot keep pace with him. In order that they can share in the same rhythm of mounting excitement and that he does not have his orgasm so long before his wife that she only reaches orgasm with difficulty, it is important that he should hold back and not allow himself to ejaculate until he can tell from the woman's breathing, the rhythmic muscular movements inside the vagina and the manner in which she embraces him, that she is sharing the same crescendo of desire and will be able to reach orgasm. Only then should he allow himself to penetrate so deep that he cannot resist ejaculating. On her part, it is important that she should help her husband to practise the self-control and patience needed to do this effectively, and that she should not make movements of so violent a nature that his excitement becomes intolerable; she should save these most passionate love movements until she knows that they are sharing the same experience and that they have caught each other's rhythm.

1. Rupert Brooke, 'Kindliness', *Collected Poems,* Sidgwick and Jackson, 1923.

When the woman has had a tear or an episiotomy which required stitching some difficulty in intercourse may be encountered at first, and she is unlikely to want to have intercourse until the repair has healed completely. I write about this very personal matter because so many women have telephoned me because they were seriously worried about this after their baby's birth, and they often do not like to mention the subject to the midwife and feel that the doctor is too busy.

The first few times a man and woman try tentative love-making after there has been an injury to the perineum, they will probably feel that it is a hopeless failure and wonder if their married life as they knew it is finished. The wife may be secretly worried and try to keep from her husband his failure to give her not only orgasm, but any degree of pleasure. She may even simulate excitement and orgasm to reassure him. It is important that a woman should be frank with her husband about this, because there are things they can do about it and because complete emotional honesty between them is a prerequisite for adjustment to each other.

The stitching is usually done at the back of the vagina and is slanted backwards and sideways, and out towards the legs. Any forceful pressure upon this part at the back of the vagina, which at first feels knobbly, rather stiff, and tender, will cause pain. If the couple desire full intercourse, any pressure should be well forward upon the front of the vagina, upon the upper ends of the inner lips and upon the base of the clitoris. The more nervous the wife that she will have pain during intercourse, the more important is it for the husband to preface entry with prolonged and tender love-play and stimulation of the erogenous zones. A warm bath with a few tablespoonfuls of ordinary kitchen salt dissolved in the water before going to bed may help considerably. The breasts may be very sensitive to touch, and all pressure upon them should be carefully avoided, as they may be tender and full, and stimulation may result in leaking of milk. The husband should concentrate upon leading his wife slowly and gently to surrender herself to him and upon delicate 'teasing' clitoral stimulation, particularly of the clitoral shaft rather than its tip. Clitoral stimulation

and clean and that they have well-balanced, carefully planned diets. If the mother's self-image is such that she demands of herself that she should live up both to the ideal of motherhood as it existed twenty or thirty years ago and also to the idea of motherhood which is currently being formed in our society, she is allowing herself to be pulled in so many directions at once that, whatever she does, she must fail; and will fall so short of what she is struggling to do that she may feel she wants to throw up the sponge entirely. The baby is cross, she is worn out and exasperated; her mother is in despair at her daughter's incompetence; the husband cannot imagine what all the fuss is about. The only possible answer to this sort of situation is to let the standards go and start to enjoy the baby.

There exists a type of mother who becomes very anxious and uncertain of herself if she has no rule to follow, no strict schedule to guide her – the sort of mother who feels she does not know how to interpret the baby's cries and that she will be feeding him until he has violent indigestion unless she follows some sort of time-table. If it will make the mother happier to feed her baby by the clock she should do so, allowing some leeway for the baby's hunger either side of the feeding time. That is, she should be prepared to feed him as much as an hour or so early if he is obviously hungry, and to leave him undisturbed if he is sleeping when the time for his feed comes round. For, as John Bowlby has said, 'What we must realize . . . is that it is not only what we do but the way that we do it which matters. Feeding on self-demand by an anxious and ambivalent mother will probably lead to far more problems than a routine regulated by the clock in the hands of one who is relaxed and happy.'

Another kind of woman establishes herself in the roles of both expectant and actual motherhood over-efficiently. Her life revolves around her abdomen and the mystical feeling she associates with pregnancy, and she may, as we have seen, refuse her husband intercourse or any sort of love play. She may lapse into invalidism as her day-to-day existence becomes more and more dominated by the baby inside her. This pre-occupation with approaching maternity may further extend itself into a possessive and exclusive attachment to her children whom she never willingly lets go. She still wants the child within her; she cannot bear to allow him his freedom, and goes to extreme lengths to ensure that she retains his love. She weeps bitterly when he is weaned, when he goes to school, and when he marries. This is the mother who

by her endless self-sacrifice, tries to ensure that the child is given no excuse for any feelings other than those of love and gratitude. This mother, who at first sight appears so loving, inevitably creates great resentment in her child by her demands for his love, and equally great guilt in him through her claims to be so good a mother that no sentiment but gratitude is justified. In behaving in this way she is of course not aware that she is seeking from her child the love, and the assurance that she is worthy of love, which she never had when she was small.[1]

The children of such deprived mothers tend to grow up over-dependent unless or until they become openly rebellious.

It is perhaps significant that this sort of motherhood seems outdated today. Seen as a social type rather than as a characteristic of individual psychopathology, it is part and parcel of a more stable family-centred culture in which the whole meaning of a woman's life was bound up with child-bearing and rearing and all her status was derived from that. It is rapidly changing in the West, although less quickly in certain Continental countries than in Britain and America. Evidently societies in which clear cultural patterns and accepted norms of behaviour are dominant and are acknowledged by large sections of the population as valid, present their problems no less than those societies which are in process of rapid cultural change.

The old traditions which formed the parent–child relationship have largely crumbled away and – since they no longer possess the validity they once had – we have to replace the custom-dominated sort of relationship, made up of a veritable jigsaw of unquestioned habitual responses and conventional patterns of behaviour, with a new perceptiveness about the quality of that relationship and the conditions under which it

1. John Bowlby, op. cit.

can best flourish. And together with this, we have to accept the instinctual ground of our being, the feelings about our children, the love and the hate that we sometimes have for them, so that we see ourselves and them with honesty. Only under such conditions is it likely that human personality can be given its greatest opportunities of development.

It seems to me that childbirth experienced with joy, in which both husband and wife share, is something valuable not only in itself but as part of the process of growth of the sort of confident motherhood and fatherhood which has its roots in happy marriage. Not all couples, of course, are capable of this. Some have made so many initial mistakes in their marriage that they find it hard – perhaps impossible – to rediscover – or to find for the first time – 'togetherness' on which to base any sort of joint preparation for parenthood. Some of the difficulties which may confront them I have touched on in the course of this book. For a large number of couples these difficulties will not be insurmountable and may in themselves constitute a challenge the accepting of which can be richly rewarding.

Parenthood does not begin with the birth of the child, nor with the germination of the seed. It has its beginnings even before the child's conception, and is part and parcel of the marriage and the love from the expression of which the baby owes his being. If this is so, our abilities as good mothers and fathers – and our failures too – cannot be viewed in isolation, apart from the sum total – the interaction and fusing of personalities – which makes up the marriage.

This is really what I mean when I call my approach to preparation for birth the Psychosexual Method: it is education not only for the pregnant woman, but for the man too, and it is concerned not only with the act of birth, but with people in a relationship of love and interdependence. Subjective experience of labour is really not just a matter of the present, but also of the past – the sort of upbringing and experiences in childhood the woman has had. It is not simply a matter of intellectual concepts and knowledge, of ideas about childbearing which are more or less accurate – but of body images rooted in infancy – which grow out of touching and being touched, and the juxtaposition and relationships of bodies.

And birth is not merely a mechanical process of getting a baby born – nor should be even if it could be achieved. It is part of a marriage, and can enrich or deprive it according to how the experience is lived through by both man and woman.

I hope to have shown in these pages how this experience can bring not only the minimum of pain and discomfort for the mother, but a deep sense of satisfaction, and exhilaration and a lasting joy for both parents.

Appendix

PREPARING FOR THE CONFINEMENT AT HOME

It is useful to get everything for the confinement prepared at least three weeks in advance and ready on a trolley or table out of sight, covered by a towel. In addition to the jam-jars (usually one for the nail-brush and one for the thermometer), bowls and news-papers which will be on the midwife's list the parents may like to have:

1 pyjama top or short nightdress for labour. Other pyjamas or nightdresses for changing into afterwards.

Dressing-gown and slippers.

Bed socks, especially when the baby is to be born in winter, so that the mother does not get chilled during labour in walking from bedroom to bathroom and back.

Extra towels and blankets, and a blanket or rug in the lavatory for throwing round the mother's shoulders in cold weather. Some safe method of quickly heating up the room before the delivery of the baby.

An electric heating pad with a plastic cover, or a couple of hot water bottles.

An electric kettle in the bedroom or a room nearby.

A tin of fruit juice and a large bottle of eau de cologne in the refrigerator.

Stick of barley sugar or sugar lumps to suck, or honey if pre-ferred, for the early first stage only.

Two small sponges to soak with iced water for refreshing the mother at the end of the first stage.

A watch or clock with a second hand if possible in the room so that the husband can time the intervals between contractions.

An extra lamp with a 100-watt bulb, and a shade which can be tilted for the delivery so that the light does not shine in the mother's eyes, or an Anglepoise type of lamp.

Three or four extra pillows for supporting the back during the second stage and possibly also the late first stage, and a large firm pillow or bolster in a polythene bag for putting under the knees so that the legs do not pull on the abdominal muscles.

A pedal bin which can be moved up to the bedroom for dirty swabs.

Disposal paper bags for soiled sanitary pads, etc. Disposable napkins. These, torn in half, and put inside each nappy, prevent excessive soiling.

Oil is needed for the baby's skin rather than dusting powder, which tends to cake up. Talc is, however, pleasant in hot weather.

Silicone cream or lanoline is useful if nipples get sore with the first feeds.

Some cakes and biscuits should be stored away in tins in advance so that one has something to offer the visitors who will come. If the mother is not having outside domestic help, but if her husband is staying at home to look after her, she should plan roughly the meals for the first three days after the birth, and see that all the ingredients are available.

The bed – preferably a single divan type without a footboard – should be pulled out from the wall if necessary when the time comes, so that there is space on both sides and at the foot of it. The mattress should be firm and is best covered with plastic or rubber sheeting. The sheet should be sufficiently large to tuck in well, or it may work loose as the mother moves. Nylon sheets and pillow cases speed up laundering during the first few days after the birth, but can be hot in summer, as a newly delivered woman tends to perspire a good deal.

A NOTE ABOUT CLASSES

The National Childbirth Trust, 9 Queensborough Terrace, London W2, can give further information about classes for expectant mothers in Sheila Kitzinger's Psychosexual Method, and about seminars and study days for midwives, physiotherapists and all antenatal teachers.

Index

Index

Where whole chapters cover subjects they have not been included again in the index, except where these subjects occur elsewhere in the book.

Titles of books, articles and journals are printed in italics, and specific exercises in bold type.

MORE ABOUT PENGUINS
AND PELICANS

Penguinews, which appears every month, contains details of all the new books issued by Penguins as they are published. From time to time it is supplemented by *Penguins in Print*, which is a complete list of all available books published by Penguins. (There are well over three thousand of these.)

A specimen copy of *Penguinews* will be sent to you free on request, and you can become a subscriber for the price of the postage. For a year's issues (including the complete lists) please send 30p if you live in the United Kingdom, or 60p if you live elsewhere. Just write to Dept EP, Penguin Books Ltd, Harmondsworth, Middlesex, enclosing a cheque or postal order, and your name will be added to the mailing list.

Note: *Penguinews* and *Penguins in Print*
are not available in the U.S.A. or Canada

CHILD CARE AND THE GROWTH OF LOVE

New Enlarged Edition

JOHN BOWLBY

In 1951, under the auspices of the World Health Organization, Dr John Bowlby wrote a report on *Maternal Care and Mental Health* which collated expert world opinion on the subject and the issues arising from it – the prevention of juvenile and adult delinquency, the problem of the 'unwanted child', the training of women for motherhood, and the best ways of supplying the needs of children deprived of their natural mothers. This book is a summary of Dr Bowlby's report, freed from many of its technicalities and prepared for the general reader.

This new edition contains chapters based on an article by Dr Mary Salter Ainsworth, written in 1962 also for the World Health Organization when it once again made an important study of child care.

'It is a convenient and scholarly summary of evidence of the effects upon children of lack of personal attention, and it presents to administrators, social workers, teachers and doctors a reminder of the significance of the family' – *The Times*

An Open University Set Book

also available:

ATTACHMENT

a Penguin Handbook

CHILDBIRTH

W. C. W. NIXON

The author of this informative handbook was Professor of Obstetrics and Gynaecology in the University of London and was director of the obstetric unit at University College Hospital from 1946.

'With every advance, scientific or sociological,' he wrote, 'the hazards of childbirth are being still further reduced. Yet there are a number of women who fear pregnancy and labour ... I believe, through personal observation, that one can face a situation much better if one knows the facts. The purpose of this book is to present some of the facts which have an important bearing on the process of birth.' This helpful account of what can be the happiest experience in a woman's life is well illustrated with diagrams (of exercises) and plates of a remarkable series of models.

THE CHILD, THE FAMILY,
AND THE OUTSIDE WORLD

D. W. WINNICOTT

Long clinical experience gave Dr Winnicott a unique standing in child psychiatry and few experts did more to present the world of children and parents to the general public.

Beginning at the natural bond between mother and child – the bond we call love, which is the key to personality – Dr Winnicott deals in turn in this volume with the phases of mother/infant, parent/child, and child/school. From the problems – which are not really problems – of feeding, weaning, and innate morality in babies, he ranges to the very real difficulties of only children, of stealing and lying, and of first experiments in independence. Shyness, sex education in schools, and the roots of aggression are among the many other topics the author covers in a book which, for its manner of imparting knowledge simply and sympathetically, must be indispensable for intelligent parents.

'His style is lucid, his manner friendly, and his years of experience provide much wise insight into child behaviour and parental attitudes' – *British Journal of Psychology*

CHILDHOOD AND ADOLESCENCE

J. A. HADFIELD

Parents in these days are often caught between distaste for Victorian strictness and mistrust of the licence which sometimes seems to be encouraged by psychologists. They no longer know when to say 'Yes' and when to say 'No' to their children.

In this new book the author of *Dreams and Nightmares* draws on a long clinical experience to describe, in simple terms, a child's natural equipment, the theory of maturation, the phases of early development, the organization of personality, and the period of adolescence. There cannot be any easy rules for rearing children and only such knowledge, therefore, can help intelligent and sympathetic parents in their dilemma.

As the author shows here, in an atmosphere of love there need be no conflict between discipline and freedom. Moreover, parents who are prepared to promote a child's mental health – in other words, the full development of its whole personality – are setting it on the right path to be successful, moral in outlook, possessed of a strong will, and as intelligent as its nature allows.

THE PSYCHOLOGY OF CHILDHOOD
AND ADOLESCENCE

C. I. SANDSTRÖM

In this concise study of the processes of growing up Professor Sandström has produced a book which, although it is perfectly suited to the initial needs of university students and teachers in training, will appeal almost as much to parents and ordinary readers. His text covers the whole story of human physical and mental growth from conception to puberty.

Outlining the scope and history of developmental psychology, Professor Sandström goes on to detail the stages of growth in the womb, during the months after birth, and (year by year) up to the age of ten. There follow chapters on physical development, learning and perception, motivation, language and thought, intelligence, the emotions, social adjustment, and personality. The special conditions of puberty and of schooling are handled in the final chapters.

Throughout this masterly study the author necessarily refers to norms of development; these neatly represent the average stages of growing up, but (as Professor Mace comments in his introduction) they must only be applied to individual children with caution.

PATTERNS OF INFANT CARE
IN AN URBAN COMMUNITY

JOHN AND ELIZABETH NEWSON

Mother, doctor, health visitor, midwife – Spock, Gibbens, de Kok, Truby King . . . the amount of theory and advice, both professional and amateur, that showers on the young mother is equalled only by its astonishing contradictions. And indeed, as the authors quietly point out, 'very few theories of child rearing have been subjected to the inconvenience of being reconciled with the empirical evidence'.

What then is that evidence? Armed with common sense and a tape recorder, the authors interviewed in their Nottingham homes over 700 mothers of one-year-old children to find out, quite simply, how babies are brought up in England today. The result is a landmark in our knowledge of childhood. The answers parents gave on subjects ranging from breast- and bottle-feeding, sleeping, eating, and punishment, to father's place in the home and class differences in infant rearing make a fascinating and, on occasions, hilarious kaleidoscope of life with young children.

'Wonderfully human piece of sociological research' – *Yorkshire Post*

THE SAFETY OF THE
UNBORN CHILD

GEOFFREY CHAMBERLAIN

The unborn child is usually perfectly safe. However, various risks are occasionally given publicity, and these often build up to become major worries to the pregnant woman. Often she feels that it would be childish and time-wasting to air these problems to others but they remain in her mind.

This book gives a straight presentation of the hazards to the unborn child, assesses them, and displays them against the background of normality. It therefore deals with material not often discussed outside the confines of the consulting room, and sometimes not discussed frankly enough even there. It is offered as a practical contribution to the understanding of pregnancy, and also in the hope of allaying many unspoken worries of pregnant women.